The Extraordinary
Healing Power
of Ordinary Things

The Extraordinary Healing Power of Ordinary Things

Fourteen Natural Steps to Health and Happiness

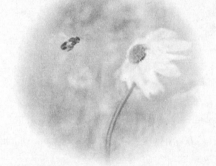

Larry Dossey, M.D.

HARMONY BOOKS • NEW YORK

Grateful acknowledgment is made to the following for permission to reprint
from these previously published works:

Alfred A. Knopf for an excerpt from *Tao Te Ching* by Lao Tsu, translated by
Gia-Fu Feng and Jane English. Translation copyright © 1997 by Jane English.
Copyright © 1972 by Gia-Fu Feng and Jane English. Reprinted by permission
of Alfred A. Knopf, a division of Random House, Inc.

Michael Grosso for an excerpt from *Soulmaking: Uncommon Paths to Self-
Understanding* by Michael Grosso. Copyright © 1997 by Michael Grosso.
Published by Hampton Roads. Used by permission of the author.

Some of the material in this book previously appeared in different
form in *Alternative Therapies in Health and Medicine*.

ISBN 0-307-20989-X

Printed in the United States of America

Design by Chris Welch

For Barbara

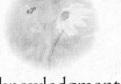

Acknowledgments

I have always been attracted to the veiled power of ordinary, commonplace things. By reasons of birth and upbringing on a spare farm in the ascetic culture of central Texas, the austere side of life has always had great appeal. To my parents I owe a debt I can never repay, because it is not possible to measure, let alone pay back, unconditional love and unstinting sacrifice. The gift is simply too great, and my resources too meager. Nonetheless, this book, which extols the greatness in "what is commonly thought small," as Virginia Woolf says, is a token of gratitude to my mother and father.

During the construction of this book, I have had the great good fortune to work with a remarkably talented editor and publisher, Toinette Lippe. When we began this collaboration, I did not know that she was the author of *Nothing Left Over: A Plain and Simple Life*, a wise book that is congruent with my premise in this one. As I sought ways of expressing the value of simplicity, she lived and painted it. Along with manuscript pages that flew back and forth, she regularly sent me electronic versions of her brushstroke art of fruit, vegetables, and flowers. These simple but elegant images reminded me to be less stuffy and verbose, yanked me back on track, and perked me up. I bow deeply.

To my literary agents, Arielle Eckstat, James Levine, and Kitty Farmer, I am grateful. A book could not have better ambassadors.

Some of these chapters had their first incarnation, in different form, in the journal *Alternative Therapies in Health and Medicine*, for which I served as executive editor for nearly a decade beginning in 1995, and to which I am grateful. Should readers be interested, I shall continue exploring the role of consciousness and spirituality in health as executive editor of *Explore: The Journal of Science and Healing (www. explorejournal.com)*.

Goethe said, "The sum which two married people owe to one another defies calculation. It is an infinite debt, which can only be discharged through all eternity." Barbara, my wife, is my greatest exemplar of extraordinariness. Because Goethe's eternity shall have to wait a while, this book is dedicated to Barbara now, in yet another unpayable debt. She appears often in these chapters, because for decades our paths have been intertwined and often indistinguishable. Our relationship has greatly influenced this book about simple things—for "simple" originally meant together, united, a whole.

Contents

Contents

If we had a keen vision of all that is ordinary in human life, it would be like hearing the grass grow or the squirrel's heart beat, and we should die of that roar which is the other side of silence.

—GEORGE ELIOT, *Middlemarch*

Examine for a moment an ordinary mind on an ordinary day.... Let us not take it for granted that life exists more fully in what is commonly thought big than in what is commonly thought small.

—VIRGINIA WOOLF, *Modern Fiction*

That's what I want to get into this book—the astonishingness of the most obvious things.

—ALDOUS HUXLEY, *Point Counter Point*

The Extraordinary
Healing Power
of Ordinary Things

Introduction

There is an old saying: If you want to hide the treasure, put it in plain sight. Then *no one* will see it.

In the pages that follow, we will explore things that are in plain sight, but whose healing power and ability to add to life's fulfillment have been overlooked or forgotten. These are ordinary, simple things. Some of them are elegant and lovely, such as music. Others seem lowly, such as dirt, or exceedingly common, such as plants. One involves, quite literally, nothing. But what they all have in common is an extraordinary capacity to help us heal, to understand our place in the natural order, and to be more complete human beings.

Modern medicine is not simple. It is increasingly complex—think genomics, stem cells, transplantation, drugs, and surgery. It often ignores those very things that can heal us, particularly if they are plain and ordinary. Unfortunately, it sometimes seems that modern medicine is actually hostile or contemptuous toward simple approaches, as if they are in some way opposed to medical science. Nothing could be further from the truth.

While we should be grateful for the high-tech, life-saving developments of modern medicine, there is a dark side to these approaches, which we ignore at our peril. Some scholars say that modern hospital care has become the third leading cause of death in America, after heart disease and cancer, because of deaths due to medical errors, mistakes, and the side effects of drugs.[1] Moreover, surveys suggest that three-fourths of those who go to doctors' offices have nothing wrong with them physically, meaning that they are largely beyond the reach of what complex, modern medicine has to offer. These facts should give us pause to ask whether there are not simpler and less lethal ways of approaching healing. I believe these ways are all around us—treasures hidden in plain sight.

We do not have to invent these measures. They already exist. They are ready to assist us when we are ready to receive their offerings. All that is required is that we approach the simple, ordinary side of the world with gratitude and respect. If we do, we may be surprised by what happens.

Although many of the chapters that follow deal specifically with health issues, others speak to health in a general sense. Health and healing are about more than the eradication of disease. *Health* is related to *wholeness* and *holy*—knowing who we are and how we are connected with the world around us. Throughout history, questions about our identity and our place in the natural order have stimulated more wonder than answers. But this is for the good because, as Aristotle said, wonder is the beginning of wisdom.

Ordinary comes from Latin and originally meant "orderly and regular."[2] *Plain* initially meant "broad, level, flat, free from obstructions," thus "open, clearly understood, evident, obvious."[3] *Simple* formerly meant "one or together, a unified whole."[4] Over time, simple came to imply that something consisted of only one part, feature, or substance; not compounded or complex; easy to do, solve, or understand.

We are drawn to simple things. Whether in art, literature, science, religion, or politics, we prefer to be spoken to directly and clearly.

Even though someone's arguments may be valid, if they are convoluted or opaque we declare him "too clever by half" and turn away. When art and architecture become excessively ornate, we regard them as decadent and we go searching for something less fussy. History's dustbin is crammed with people, ideas, and movements that were marginalized and forgotten because the originators thought clarity a vice.

The deadliest temptation of artists and writers is to be deeply profound—deadly because this often leads to byzantine, impenetrable complexity. Unless they manage to escape this trap, their work seldom endures. Thus, the French novelist and essayist Stendahl: "I see but one rule: to be clear. If I am not clear, all my world crumbles to nothing."[5]

Even in science, which laypersons often consider hopelessly complex, simplicity is accorded a high value. One of science's guiding tenets is Ockham's razor, formulated by William of Ockham (c. 1300–c. 1349). This "principle of parsimony" states that simple explanations should be preferred to complicated ones.

But simple things can also mislead us, because what seems simple often conceals an intricacy that is not obvious. When I visit an art museum and view a famous painting, I often think, "I could do that!" But immediately another voice kicks in, reminding me that great art is not as simple as it seems. Nowhere is this more obvious than in the Japanese arts of painting, calligraphy, and flower arranging. An ikebana floral arrangement may look simple, and it is—but try doing it! A single-brushstroke apple may appear to be achievable by any kindergarten student, but it can be maddeningly difficult. Great lives, like great art, are always more complex than they seem. A joke among the wealthy supporters of the ascetic Mahatma Gandhi during India's struggle for independence from Great Britain was that it took a fortune to keep him in poverty. So too in science. Einstein's $E = mc^2$ is one of the simplest equations in physics, but nested within it are concepts that are bewilderingly complex and counterintuitive. Einstein realized this, of course, and tried to wave off those who didn't.

"Things should be made as simple as possible," he once said, "but not any simpler."[6]

Why do simple, ordinary things attract us? Cynics say it is because we are lazy or incompetent; we don't want to expend the mental effort required to engage the complex, or we don't possess the intellectual firepower required to do so—thus the "dumbing down" that is epidemic in contemporary life. I believe otherwise. The primary reason we are drawn to the simple and the ordinary is contained in the original meaning of simple: one, a unity, a whole. Simplicity and ordinariness remind us of what Buddhists call our original nature—our unbroken wholeness with the All, the Absolute, the Divine, however it is named. Our innate preference for the simple is then a spiritual tug—not a descent into indolence, but an ascent to transcendent oneness.

Our culture urges the individual to stand out, to be unique and extraordinary. I have always been fascinated by Native American cultures that took a different view. In them, fitting into the social fabric, not standing out, was considered the supreme achievement. From the individual's dedication to the tribe, high accomplishments and uniqueness often arose naturally, revealing that the ordinary and the extraordinary are not opposed.

But we should not romanticize the plain. Although the best things in life are usually simple, all simple things are not good. As Tolstoy says in "The Death of Ivan Ilych," "Ivan Ilych's life had been most simple and most ordinary and therefore most terrible."[7] Consider manual labor. Any Third World woman who has performed the quite ordinary act of carrying water for miles before breakfast prefers the more complicated situation of a faucet inside her hut. Any farmer who has toiled for years at the end of a hoe deems a mechanical device that lessens his work heaven-sent. My goal is therefore not to idealize simple things, but to focus on the variety of simplicities that *can* bring healing and fulfillment to our lives, and which often do.

Agreement on the virtues of simplicity is hard to come by. When the legendary modernist architect Mies van der Rohe said, "Less is more,"[8] he was satirized by post-modernist architect Robert Venturi with, "Less is a bore."[9] Perhaps what follows will provoke similar disagreement—unless you, dear reader, bear in mind that opposites complement one another and are not antithetical.

The most profound healing event I remember was being touched by a nurse when I was recovering from anesthesia following an appendectomy. The surgery was a rushed-up affair that took place in the Student Health Center at the University of Texas-Austin while I was preparing to enter medical school. I never met the surgeon beforehand; he thought it unnecessary. When I awoke, I was anxious, alone, and in pain. The nurse's lingering touch conveyed to me—silently, powerfully, unequivocally—that everything was going to be all right. It was, and the occasion is seared into my memory. I've been hooked on simple, ordinary health interventions ever since.

Now let's listen to the plainsong of healing.

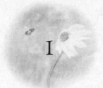

Optimism

A pessimist asks you if there is milk in the pitcher;
an optimist asks you to pass the cream.

—*FOLK SAYING*

It troubles me to recall him even now, many years later—the fifty-year-old attorney who gave me my most painful lesson in the value of optimism and what happens when it fades away. He was at the peak of his career, father of three, athletic, a picture of health. His only concern was a minor stomachache that had come and gone for a couple of weeks. Even though his physical examination was normal, he insisted on an abdominal scan just to be sure nothing was wrong. Although I thought this overkill, I went along. To my surprise, the scan showed a mass in the pancreas the radiologist said was probably cancer. I discussed the situation with him and proposed a diagnostic workup, including the possibility of eventual abdominal surgery. "No surgery!" he declared emphatically. "It's worthless. Nobody survives cancer of the pancreas." I pointed out that he was mistaken. Although the statistics are not favorable, people do survive this disease. In any case, we weren't sure of the diagnosis and further tests were needed to confirm it.

He consented to be hospitalized that very day, but a light went out in him. He seemed terrified, and nothing I could say would comfort him. He began to stare straight ahead, refusing to speak to me or the nurses. When I made rounds that evening, he lay silent and rigid in bed with clenched jaws and furrowed brow. Even when I informed him that his preliminary blood tests were normal, he didn't seem to care. In his mind he was a condemned man going to the gallows. I resolved that if his behavior did not change by morning, I would ask a psychiatrist to consult on his case. I didn't get the chance. That night the nurse found him dead in bed.

His was a "hex death," widely recognized in premodern cultures, in which a previously healthy individual dies shortly after being cursed. The curse—in this case, his certainty that he had a fatal illness—removes all optimism and hope, and substitutes the inevitability of death.[1]

Optimism is the tendency to believe, expect, or hope that things will turn out well. Debates have raged over the past few years about whether it affects our health and the course of specific diseases. I find these arguments tedious, because I believe evidence of the healing power of optimism is in plain sight. These effects are most obvious when they vary from day to day, like shifting winds. In the 1950s, Dr. Bruno Klopfer reported such an example that involved a patient he was treating for advanced lymphoma. The man had large tumors throughout his body and fluid in his chest, and was terminal. Klopfer was so convinced that he would die within two weeks that all medical therapy except oxygen had been discontinued. In a last-ditch effort he gave the man a single injection of Krebiozen, an experimental drug later said to be worthless. Klopfer describes the results:

What a surprise was in store for me! I had left him febrile, gasping for air, completely bedridden. Now, here he was, walking around the ward, chatting happily with the nurses, and spreading his message of good cheer to anyone who would listen. . . . The tumor masses had melted like snow balls on a hot stove,

and in only these few days they were half their original size!
This is, of course, far more rapid regression than the most
radiosensitive tumor could display under heavy x-ray given every
day. . . . And he had no other treatment outside of the single
useless "shot."

Within ten days the man was practically free of disease. He began
to fly his private airplane again. His improvement lasted for two
months, until reports cropped up denouncing Krebiozen. When he
read them, the man appeared cursed, and his attitude and medical
condition quickly returned to a terminal state. At this point Klopfer
urged the man to ignore the negative news reports because a "new
super-refined, double-strength product" was now available—a complete fabrication—and injected him with sterile water. The man's
response this time was even more dramatic than initially, and he
resumed his normal activities for another two months. But his
improvement ended when the American Medical Association released
a report stating that nationwide tests had proved Krebiozen useless in
the treatment of cancer. A few days after reading this statement, he
was admitted to the hospital, and two days following admission
he died.[2]

If optimism can make such dramatic differences, you'd think we
physicians would do everything in our power to increase it in our
patients, but sometimes we seem hell-bent on depriving them of it.
Some of these instances are so outrageous they are almost funny.

Andrew Weil, MD, who is director of the program in integrative
medicine at the University of Arizona in Tucson, often sees patients
for a second opinion.[3] "You wouldn't believe what those doctors did
to me," one woman related. "The head neurologist took me into his
office and told me I had multiple sclerosis. He let that sink in; then
he went out of the room and returned with a wheelchair. Then he
told me to sit in it. I said, 'Why should I sit in your wheelchair?' He
said I was to buy a wheelchair and sit in it for an hour a day to 'practice' for when I would be totally disabled. Can you imagine?"

In his book *The Lost Art of Healing,* Harvard cardiologist Bernard Lown gives examples of "words that maim" by depriving patients of optimism and hope. They include, "You are living on borrowed time," "You are going downhill fast," "The next heartbeat may be your last," "You can have a heart attack or worse any minute," "The . . . angel of death . . . is shadowing you," "You are a walking time bomb," "I'm frightened just thinking about your [coronary] anatomy," and "Surgery should be done immediately, preferably yesterday."[4] To these medical hexes, Weil adds a few more: "They said there was nothing more they could do for me," "They told me it would only get worse," "They told me I would just have to live with it," and "They said I'd be dead in six months."[5]

Why do we physicians find it so difficult to accord optimism a role in health? Why is it so hard for us to be optimistic? You might think we'd be positively euphoric, because we have more potent tools in our black bags than ever before, and the human lifespan is at an all-time high. Why aren't we joyful? The fact is, physicians are trained to be realists, not optimists, and our realism often shades into pessimism. The specter of death hangs over every clinical encounter, a shadow that never goes away no matter how powerful our therapies become. We know that all our treatments will eventually fail and the patient will die; never has there been an exception. Thus the beginning assumption of medicine is tragedy. No other profession rests on such a morbid foundational belief. This is why it is so natural for a physician to be a pessimist, and why optimism is the hard thing.

Pessimism dominates some physicians and colors everything they do. I've known physicians who actually cultivate cynicism and take pride in a morose, gloomy personal style. Some wear their pessimism as a badge of honor. This often involves what's called "hanging crepe"—black crepe, as at a funeral—in which the physician emphasizes the worst possible outcome of any situation. If the prophecy comes true, the physician is wise; if not, he is a hero, having rescued his patient from his dire predictions.

It is unethical, we are taught, to paint a rosy future for a patient who is facing a grave health challenge when we know the outcome is likely to be the opposite. The problem, however, is that the physician's realism can trigger disastrous results. Consider medical prognosis. When a physician tells a patient she has a fifty percent chance of *living* twelve months, the patient is likely to interpret this as a fifty percent chance of *dying* by the end of a year. The patient, failing to understand that the doctor is simply making a calculated guess, often converts the statistical prediction into a death sentence by dying on schedule.

But it is never only a matter of the words that a physician uses to deliver bad news, it's also how they are conveyed. Some physicians are able to express bad news with such compassion that the sense of impending tragedy is annulled. How do they do it? The way physicians always have—through deep empathy and caring for those they serve. They convey a sense of love and oneness with their patient, as if to say, "Together we will do our best. No matter what happens, I am with you every step of the way; you will never be alone."

If profound pessimism can kill, why is it so widespread? Why would evolution have permitted it to persist? What purpose would pessimism have served? "The benefits of pessimism," suggests psychologist Martin E. P. Seligman, former president of the American Psychological Association and author of *Learned Optimism*, "may have arisen during our recent evolutionary history. We are animals of the Pleistocene, the epoch of the ice ages. Our emotional makeup has most recently been shaped by one hundred thousand years of climatic catastrophe: waves of cold and heat; drought and flood; plenty and sudden famine. Those of our ancestors who survived the Pleistocene may have done so because they had the capacity to worry incessantly about the future, to see sunny days as mere prelude to a harsh winter, to brood. We have inherited these ancestors' brains and therefore their capacity to see the cloud rather than the silver lining."[6]

The survival value of pessimism may date from the era when humans descended from treetops onto the savannas of Africa. These open grasslands were the home of the great stalking cats and were dangerous places. Pessimism would have lent an edge in the struggle to survive—not pessimism that overwhelmed and drove our ancestors back into the safety of the forests, but enough to guarantee wariness and survival.

But perhaps we should not concede too much to pessimism. It is difficult to imagine how *Homo sapiens* could have advanced from savage to barbarian to civilization without a sense that things might be better. How could we have journeyed from caves to castles, from skins to silks, from dominance to democracy, without optimism? Without the beckoning light of a brighter future, it would have been easy to quit in the early days and settle for the status quo. Something kept us going toward a dawn not fully glimpsed, and optimism is as good a name as any for this indwelling itch.

Ultimate Optimism

It's easy to be optimistic about optimism these days. Research shows that optimists on average get sick less often and live longer than pessimists. The immune system seems to be stronger in optimists, and the cardiovascular system more stable. Optimists are the go-getters, achievers, and leaders who are held high in public esteem. Optimists are generally likable; they pump others up, and people enjoy their company more than that of pessimists. There is a new field, positive psychology, that stresses the value of optimism. Optimism is so hot it recently made the cover of *Time* magazine.[7]

Optimism is on a roll—and I sometimes feel as if it is about to roll over me. Although I am personally inclined toward optimism, I tremble at the showy, smiley-faced, shotgun variety that is advocated these days by the insufferable optimism merchants. I favor a quiet, indwelling variety of optimism that I keep to myself as a calm certainty. I hesitate to name this attitude; even calling it a "cognitive style," as the positive psychologists do, is going too far. As Stendahl said about happiness, "To describe [it] is to diminish it."[8] My approach is akin to what medieval theologians called the *via negativa*, the negative way, which emphasized the fullness and reality of the Divine by dwelling not on positive attributes, but on the fact that the Divine is beyond description. Attributing any quality to the Absolute was a form of anthropomorphic idolatry, dressing up the godhead in human form. Meister Eckhart, the thirteenth-century German mystic, was a proponent of the *via negativa*. He said, "Then how shall I love him?—Love him as he is: a not-God, a not-spirit, a not-Person, a not-image; as sheer, pure, limpid unity, alien from all duality. And in this one let us sink down eternally from nothingness to nothingness. So help us God. Amen."[9] In keeping with Eckhart's view, perhaps I should call my attitude not-optimism.

For me, linking optimism and the Absolute or Divine, however named, is not hyperbole. The connection is natural: *Optimism* comes from Latin words meaning "highest" or "best," which is what we consider the Divine to be. Julian of Norwich, England's sublime fourteenth-century mystic, understood this relationship. At a time when the Black Death was stalking Europe, she found no difficulty associating optimism and the Divine. In enchanting prose she exulted, "But all shall be well, and all shall be well, and all manner of thing shall be well . . . He said not 'Thou shalt not be tempested, thou shalt not be travailed, thou shalt not be diseased,' but he said, 'Thou shalt not be overcome' "[10] Or as poet Maya Angelou has echoed in our day, "You may encounter many defeats, but you must not be defeated."[11]

Optimism unanchored to the Absolute is hard to sustain. If one takes the distant view of modern cosmology, the scenario is bottomlessly depressing. Our expanding universe, scientists tell us, will eventually undergo heat death and will descend into irreversible disorganization. This means that life and consciousness will perish. Against this backdrop, optimism is a worthless, pitiful Band-Aid. But if consciousness is linked with the Absolute, the outlook changes. The Absolute stands above all, including whatever may happen to the cosmos. Our connectedness with the Absolute implies that we share qualities with it—qualities which, much evidence suggests,[12] include infinitude in space and time. If so, we are in some sense eternal and immortal: the ultimate justification for being optimistic, and a finger in the eye of doomsaying cosmologists.

Exuberance: Profound Optimism

In some people optimism shades into exuberance, a sense of overflowing joy and energy. Kay Redfield Jamison, the psychiatrist who made headlines in exposing her own bipolar illness,[13] has written a book, *Exuberance: The Passion for Life*, which includes interviews with many exuberant people.[14] Everyone she interviewed described how annoying they could be to others. Highly optimistic, exuberant people are also easily annoyed by others; many of those in very competitive environments such as universities and research institutions where objectivity is in demand said they felt very vulnerable to ridicule.

One reason exuberant people are resented by their colleagues is that they make others uncomfortable after a certain point. As Jamison says, "They like being around them, enjoy the energy and the enthusiasm, but it is kind of exhausting." Or as the author Elbert Hubbard (1856–1915) said, "A pessimist is a man who has been compelled to live with an optimist."[15]

Unrestrained exuberance can also be hazardous. Jamison again: "We all need to have . . . skepticism about ourselves. Exuberance can be dangerous. If you have someone who is exuberant and doing great and wonderful things, that is terrific. But if you have somebody who is leading you into war because he or she is very enthusiastic about it, or into very bad business deals. . . ."[16]

Optimism Tested, Optimism Twisted

Optimism was repeatedly put to the test during the twentieth century with two world wars, the Holocaust, repeated genocides, and a death toll unparalleled in any era. Challenges to optimism are continuing into the twenty-first century.

On December 26, 2004, an earthquake on the sea floor off Sumatra generated a monstrous tsunami that lashed coastlines as far away as Africa, killing an estimated 150,000 individuals. Entire families and whole villages vanished. Hearts around the world ached for the victims and, in another kind of flood, millions of dollars of aid poured in from governments and individuals everywhere.

The disaster generated around-the-clock news coverage in which pundits tried to find meaning in the disaster. These programs featured agnostics, atheists, scientists, philosophers, statesmen, politicians, and clerics of various religions. The agnostics, atheists, and scientists generally saw the tsunami as an expression of the blind laws of nature—"nature red in tooth and claw." To them, there was no essential meaning to the event, because the laws of nature, they believe, are coldly impersonal and inherently meaningless. In contrast, several Islamic commentators managed to find positive meaning and optimism in the event. They said that the Christians, Jews, and Westerners who perished at seaside resorts were infidels and heretics who deserved their heaven-sent punishment. As Saudi cleric Muhammad al-Munajjid said in an interview on Saudi/UAE's Al-Majd TV, "Haven't they [Western tourists celebrating Christmas holidays] learned the lesson from what Allah wreaked upon the coast of Asia, during the celebration of these forbidden [festivals]? At the height of immorality, Allah took vengeance on these criminals." But what of the thousands of Muslims who died alongside the infidels? They were considered martyrs.[17] It was a sorry moment. Optimism, in the hands of religion, can take alarming forms.

These comments illustrate an eternal problem with optimism: What seems optimistic to one individual can be disastrous for another. Even in matters of health, things are clouded. All mothers, for example, want their newborns to be well and never to get sick. Yet the only way infants develop immune systems capable of resisting infections is through repeated exposures to swarms of microbes that stimulate mini-illnesses and the production of antibodies. If the hopes of the optimistic mom were realized, her child would wind up a "bubble baby" who must live inside a plastic shield to ward off the myriad bacteria, fungi, and viruses that are a part of daily life.

Another widespread expression of optimism is the hope or belief that we will recover from any illness that may strike us. If this universal wish were realized, no one would die, and the earth would have become disastrously overpopulated millennia ago and rendered unfit for human habitation.

The most egregious abuses of optimism, however, take place on a large scale and in full view. The entire advertising sector is driven by a strategy of faux optimism: your life will be happier, sexier, and better if you buy a particular product, whether or not you actually need it or can afford it. Similarly, the self-help industry also rests on a doctrine of cheery optimism and happy outcomes, if the strategy of the month is followed. And politics oscillates crazily between optimism and pessimism, each political party painting the other as pessimistic, retro, and out of touch, and itself as forward-looking, creative, and positive about the future.

Pessimism's Paradox

Pessimism, if carried to the extreme, often undergoes a weird transformation and becomes funny. This is the sort of thing that occurs in gallows humor, in which "things are so bad I might as well laugh."

Many comic geniuses understand keenly that pessimism can morph into humor, and they use this to great effect. It is no accident that some of our greatest comedians have been self-styled pessimists, such as Charlie Chaplin, W. C. Fields, Red Skelton, and Rodney Dangerfield.

Even when people try to be genuinely pessimistic, they often come off as funny and we laugh at them through their seriousness. Consider Henry Miller's put-down of optimism and hope: "Hope is a bad thing. It means that you are not what you want to be. It means that part of you is dead, if not *all* of you. It means that you entertain illusions. It's a sort of spiritual clap, I should say."[18] Or the curmudgeon who said, "Life is a sexually transmitted disease with a one hundred percent fatality rate." Or Baron de Montesquieu, who said, in all seriousness, "A man should be mourned at his birth, not at his death."[19]

If we are trapped in pessimism, perhaps we should not hold back, but plunge in and be *seriously* pessimistic, nothing halfway. If we did so we might wind up laughing, and liberate ourselves from pessimism's grasp.

The Health Connection

One of the most significant breakthroughs in twentieth-century medicine was the discovery of the importance of attitudes, emotions, and beliefs in health—what is now called mind-body medicine. Prior to mid-century, it was decidedly odd to hear clinicians speak of such things; now it is commonplace. The key premise of mind-body medicine is that our mental life is not isolated above the clavicles. Each thought and emotion is a message to the rest of the body, mediated by an intricate array of nerve signals, hormones, and various other substances.

A major development was the findings of behavioral scientists Suzanne Kobasa and Salvatore Maddi, then at the University of Chicago. In a series of landmark studies in the early 1980s, they elaborated the idea of psychological hardiness—a behavioral pattern found in stressed individuals who almost never got sick and lived long, fulfilling lives. The key, they found, was the "3 Cs"—Control, Commitment to work, family, and self, and a strong sense of Challenge. Even during periods of intense psychological stress, individuals possessing these traits remained healthy, while those who had low hardiness scores had significantly poorer health.

Kobasa and Maddi observed that the critical starting point for hardiness and effective coping is an "optimistic appraisal" of a situation. When an event is viewed with less pessimism, its psychological and physiological impact is reduced. They concluded that hardiness, effective coping, and optimism are not fixed but are flexible.

A sense of control is largely a belief one can either reject or adopt and cultivate. As Blair Justice, professor of psychology at the School of Public Health, University of Texas-Houston, says in his admirable survey of the mind-body field, *Who Gets Sick: How Beliefs, Moods, and Thoughts Affect Your Health,* "Cognitive control stems from the belief that we can affect the hurtful impact . . . of a situation by how we look at the problem. It means that by choosing to regard losses, hurts, frustrations and stressful life changes with less gloom and doom and not as the end of the world, we control their power to damage us."[20]

In study after study, people who were most resistant to physical and mental illness used a style of coping in which they viewed their situation with less pessimism. This led to taking action, where possible, to change the external problem. Then the individuals usually palliated the physical and mental effects of the stress through exercise, relaxation training, or some other healthy behavior.[21]

"Optimistic appraisal" is simply a good attitude or upbeat approach to a given situation. Lawrence Hinkle and his colleagues at New York Hospital-Cornell Medical Center followed several populations over twenty years, looking for evidence that optimistic appraisal makes a difference in health.[22] One group was a hundred Chinese immigrants who were marooned in the United States because of political unrest in their homeland. Their lives were in upheaval—uncertain about their fate and that of their families back home, and how they would survive economically. Those who remained healthy—and many did—were distinguished by how they viewed their difficulties. They saw their past and present as difficult but also interesting, challenging, and relatively satisfying. Those who got sick more often took a different view, seeing their situation as threatening, frustrating, and demanding.[23]

Hinkle and his coworkers also found that in trying circumstances there is another way to promote good health that does not involve optimism. If one insulates oneself emotionally, invests little in life, and builds walls to keep others out, the incidence of illness is also reduced.[24] But there is a downside to this approach. As Justice says in an understatement, "[O]ur social health will suffer and our relations with others will have no depth."[25]

Cardiologist Daniel B. Mark, of Duke University School of Medicine, followed the progress of 1,719 men and women after cardiac catheterization. After one year, 12 percent of people who were initially pessimistic about their health had died, compared to only 5 percent of the optimists. Dr. Nancy Frasure-Smith, of the Montreal Heart Institute, found that heart patients who scored high on pessimism were eight times more likely than optimists to die over the course of eighteen months. Dr. Geoffrey Reed, of the University of California–Los Angeles, showed that fatalism, optimism's polar opposite, and the loss of friends predicted negative outcomes in patients with HIV disease.[26]

How does optimism actually foster longer and healthier lives? Seligman suggests four ways.[27] First, the brain registers the experience of optimism and reaches down via humoral, chemical, and nerve pathways to affect cellular function throughout the body, including the cardiac, immune, and other systems. Second, because optimism is correlated with motivation and taking action, optimistic people are more likely to *want* to be healthy and to believe they *can* be healthy. This makes it more likely that they will follow healthy regimens and medical advice. Third, optimists experience fewer noxious events in their lives than pessimists, including fewer threats to their health, because their sense of control assures them that they can make a difference in what happens. In contrast, pessimists often seem to roll out a red carpet for chaos, convinced that what they do doesn't matter. Finally, optimists enjoy greater social support than pessimists, and evidence shows that even mild social interaction is a buffer against illness.[28]

Cardiologist Dean Ornish, who pioneered the reversal of heart disease by diet, exercise, and stress management, emphasizes the value of love in health. Love is perhaps the most profound type of social interaction. In his book *Love and Survival,* he suggests that our very survival depends on the healing power of love, intimacy, and relationships.[29] The link to optimism is direct: Love leads to optimism and empowers it. Optimists are more lovable than pessimistic curmudgeons, and the love they receive generates more optimism—and so on, in a self-reinforcing cycle.

Optimism is also essential to the actual practice of medicine—not as an optional nicety, but as a vital factor. Consider the placebo response, which is the sense of benefit a patient feels that arises solely from the knowledge that some treatment has been given. Researchers estimate that the placebo response accounts for 30 to 50 percent of the effect of many drugs, and sometimes up to 100 percent of certain surgical procedures.[30] All physicians know that the placebo response is an indispensable part of modern medicine, and that a good physician must know how to maximize it. The driving force behind the placebo response is optimism—the belief that the therapy will work. Optimism, therefore, in the guise of placebo effects, remains an essential part of the foundation of medicine, as it has been throughout history. But let's not forget that the placebo response has a dark twin, the nocebo effect, which is a negative and sometimes fatal result based on pessimism—the belief that a therapy will *not* work.

Barriers to Optimism

Many people find it difficult to be optimistic about their health as they age. The attention given these days to Alzheimer's disease, arthritis, and other degenerative ailments makes people see their future as a one-way ticket to a nursing home, disability, and senility. Yet there are valid grounds for optimism. Of those 65 to 74 years old, 89 percent report no disability. After age 85, 40 percent of individuals are fully functional.[31] In recent years, the percentage of people over 65 years old who are disabled has dropped, and experts predict this trend will accelerate.[32]

A wealth of evidence suggests that the choices we make about diet, weight, exercise, and social and mental stimuli during middle age greatly affect our psychological and physical competence as we age.[33] Spiritual and religious involvement are believed to add seven or more years, on average, to one's lifespan.[34] Several studies show that what one *thinks* about one's health is one of the most accurate predictors of longevity ever discovered.[35]

Many individuals find it difficult to be optimistic about their health because they come from short-lived, unhealthy families. They feel cursed by their genes, betrayed by their DNA. But, says Justice, "[G]enes account for about 35 percent of longevity, while lifestyles, diet, and other environmental factors, including support systems, are the major reasons people live longer."[36,37]

Another barrier to remaining optimistic about aging is that close friends and family members die, and we feel increasingly alone. The periodic mourning and bereavement that comes with aging are legitimate health concerns, because evidence shows that bereavement is associated with a drastic decline in immune function, which may be one reason for the increase in infections and cancer with aging.[38] It is important to mourn one's losses, and bereavement should not be short-circuited. Yet we should help bereaved individuals move *through* their mourning, and, to the extent possible, focus on life's brighter facets—not just because it is humane to assist them in this way, but also because it is healthy for them as well. Why healthy? Optimism counters the negative effects of pessimism on immune function in the elderly. In men and women between ages 62 and 87, researchers at the University of Pennsylvania found that optimistic individuals had higher helper/suppressor T-cell ratios, meaning greater ability to resist disease.[39] Other researchers found that elderly individuals who remained alive at the end of an eight-year period were those with the most optimism.[40]

Optimism: The Dark Side

Psychologist Roy Baumeister, author of *Evil: Inside Human Violence and Cruelty*,[41] and his colleagues at Case Western Reserve University explored what happens when individuals are too optimistic about themselves.[42] They examined self-esteem in serial killers, hit men, gang leaders, violent criminals, spouse abusers, and bullies. It is commonly assumed that people drift into criminality because they think poorly of themselves, but the researchers found the opposite: these individuals have enormously high levels of self-esteem. This creates in them a sense of grandiosity, supremacy, invulnerability, and the belief that they should not be corrected. When others object to their behavior, they lash out. Baumeister states, "Today, it is common to propose that low self-esteem causes violence, but the evidence shows plainly that this idea is false. This is true across a broad spectrum of violence, from play-ground bullying to national tyranny, from domestic abuse to genocide, from warfare to murder and rape. Perpetrators of violence are typically people who think very highly of themselves[43] . . . In the United States the push to raise everyone's self-esteem seems ill-advised. . . . "[44]

Optimism about the self, then, is no panacea and can be danger-ous. Boosting self-esteem indiscriminately in some youngsters may lead to disaster. You may get an egotistical kid who grows up to abuse his wife, or at worst commit a schoolyard shooting spree.[45]

Cultivating Optimism

Optimism is not a given. It can fluctuate, like our body weight, and can be learned. In his book *Learned Optimism*, psychologist Seligman shows how.[46]

It's a matter of ABC, Seligman explains. When we encounter Adversity, we begin to think about it. Over time, these thoughts ossify into Beliefs, which can become so habitual they are unconscious. Our beliefs about adverse situations have Consequences, causing us to respond either optimistically or pessimistically.

Seligman teaches people to become aware of their habitual, automatic behaviors and to substitute more adaptive, optimistic responses. Here's a typical exercise. Allow yourself to vividly imagine an everyday adversity, "A"—someone has squeezed into the parking space you were eyeing. Next, you identify the thoughts and beliefs, "B," that you have about this situation. You then imagine the consequences, "C," of these beliefs, such as honking your horn, shaking your fist, or yelling. Seligman adds a "D" and "E": Disputation, in which you engage in self-dialogue or analysis of the situation (I don't own the parking spot; others are available); and Energization, in which you seek an optimistic perspective (the driver of the other car was elderly; she needed the parking spot more than I do; giving it up is an act of kindness; I feel better having done it). Seligman advocates keeping a journal of ABCDE exercises to help jostle the mind out of habitual, pessimistic responses.

These methods have been used in children, college students, and adults. They appear capable of generating not only optimism, but positive physical changes as well. In patients with cancer, for example, sharp increases in immune function have been observed in participants using these techniques.[47,48]

Pessimists often resist methods like these because they sound gimmicky, and because they disdain efforts by optimists to convert them. Pessimists are often convinced that they "see the world aright," as the cantankerous pessimist Ambrose Bierce put it; why should they trade in their perspective for rose-colored glasses? Perhaps the most concrete reason is that optimists, research shows, get sick less often and live longer than pessimists, and that optimists are happier.

A Larger View

Henry Dreher, the science and health writer, is a keen analyst of mind-body research. In his important book *Mind-Body Unity*, he offers a stinging critique of nearly all the research touting optimism.[49] In his opinion, it's not enough to demonstrate that optimism makes a difference in health; one must also ask why it does so. Almost none of the researchers in this field, Dreher says, has asked why some sick people are optimistic, while others are pessimistic. The research specifically ignores the social factors that spawn and nourish optimism or pessimism. The result of disregarding these external factors, he believes, is that optimism is converted into a purely psychological issue. As a consequence, researchers tend to "put the onus on individuals to lift themselves out of the muck of negativism by their cognitive bootstraps." Sometimes this is successful, as in the therapies advocated by Seligman. "But," Dreher laments, "the other part of the task, the creation of neighborhoods and workplaces that generate optimism and self-efficacy, remains nearly absent from mind-body intervention research."[50]

Dreher should be listened to. He spent two years as a reading teacher in an after-school day-care program in New York City's notorious Hell's Kitchen. Most of his students lived in terrible, demoralized neighborhoods overrun with poverty and drugs. Dreher was often baffled by his students. "I was struck," he relates, "by the children who came from the worst imaginable homes and neighborhoods and yet possessed a maturity and resilience that I could not explain . . . [T]hey had psychospiritual qualities—whether from genes, early experiences, or unknown influences—that enabled them to survive." But not all were that durable. Dreher emerged from these experiences convinced that optimism was about more than psychology. He is convinced that unless researchers expand their vision to include social and economic factors, optimism research will be squeezed into "a one-sided preoccupation with getting people to change their inner lives as a cure for every ailment of mind and body."[51]

Many lab experiments show that if animals such as rats, mice, and dogs are shocked repeatedly, they lie down in their cages and give up if they do not have a way of turning off the shocks. Many people in our society, says Dreher, such as the chronically unemployed, the disaffected, and those who are discriminated against, are like the animals in these studies, unable to "turn off the shocks." Is it appropriate to ask these individuals to *think* themselves out of their plight? Dreher concludes, "[W]hile Seligman's cognitive therapy is undoubtedly helpful for many individuals, as well as for more privileged people, more is needed. . . . Yes, people can improve their lot by thinking, feeling, and behaving in more adaptive ways. But if people are asked to take greater responsibility for their attitudes and health, the social engineers, the politicians, the powerbrokers, and the medical establishment must also be asked to take greater responsibility for conditions that sometimes crush even the most resilient personalities."[52]

Health psychologist Blair Justice agrees: "When people grow up in poverty or are the victims of injustice, when they struggle day by day just to survive, their thoughts and beliefs cannot help but be deeply influenced by their environment. In the absence of love, support, minimum opportunity and security, faith and optimism are much harder to come by. By redressing wrongs and improving human conditions, we can give more people a decent chance to adopt less pessimistic views and contribute to their own health."[53] Psychiatrist Redford Williams and historian Virginia Williams, of Duke University Medical Center, support this view: "[T]he health of entire populations—nations and states—can suffer when societal relationships deteriorate . . . for example, in the widening gap between haves and have-nots."[54]

The Future of Optimism

Research linking health and longevity with socioeconomic status is so firmly established that in 2000, Justice predicted, "We can expect in the next decade considerable national debate on health policies that will focus more on strengthening low-income families, bringing more of a sense of community to neighborhoods and a sense of belonging to all within the United States. Also, policies are likely to be proposed that would result in reducing the wide gap between those on top and those on bottom in terms of income and education."[55]

Sadly, Justice's prophecy has not come to pass. The gap between rich and poor in the United States is widening. Concern about the social determinants of health is taking a back seat to glamorous, expensive interventions such as DNA and genome manipulation, stem cells, organ transplants, and new drugs.

A wave of cynicism toward the disadvantaged seems to be settling over our nation, which makes it difficult to engage the social determinants of health. The tendency is to blame people for being poor or disadvantaged, or to otherwise ignore, redefine, and obfuscate the problem. In one of his cartoons, Jules Feiffer satirized this situation: "I used to think I was poor. Then they told me I wasn't poor, I was needy. They told me it was self-defeating to think of myself as needy, I was deprived. Then they told me underprivileged was overused. I was disadvantaged. I still don't have a dime. But I have a great vocabulary."[56]

Politicians romanticize poverty by exaggerating their humble beginnings (they never brag about their privilege and wealth). Another ploy is to invoke the idea in physics of "order out of chaos"—the pretense that chaos at the social level generates order, as it often does in purely physical systems. But as John W. Gardner observed in his book *Excellence*, "For every talent that poverty has stimulated, it has blighted a hundred."[57]

Although individuals can learn optimism, as we've seen, they can also learn pessimism—as they do any time we foster social conditions that make it more difficult for people to climb out of poverty, acquire an education, and support their families. Until we take seriously the plight of the vulnerable in our nation—not just the poor but all those who find themselves the objects of every sort of prejudice and discrimination—we have no right to preach to them the virtues of optimism. Until we help change the conditions that cause pessimism, our exhortations to look on the bright side will ring hollow—for, to the seriously disadvantaged, the light we perceive at the end of the tunnel is for them an oncoming train.[58]

"A hungry man is not a free man," Adlai E. Stevenson said in 1952.[59] Neither is he an optimistic one. Who can be comfortable in their optimism when increasing numbers of our elderly must choose each day between medicine and food? When one in seven people around the world suffer from hunger, and forty million people starve to death each year or die from hunger-related diseases? When forty million are living with AIDS? When twelve million die each year from lack of water, and 1.1 billion have no access to clean water?[60] When each day in Africa alone three thousand children under the age of five die of malaria, and six thousand adults of AIDS?[61]

We must work toward an optimism that is suitable not only for the wealthy, but also for the poor, the disadvantaged, the vulnerable. Until then, we can advocate optimism only with hesitation, knowing that it has an elitist connotation we desperately need to eliminate.

In the end, it will not be weekend conferences, seminars, Web-based courses, or books that will teach people how to be optimistic; rather, it will be what we do as a nation to create the conditions in which optimism can flower.

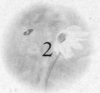

2

Forgetting

In the practical use of our intellect,
forgetting is as important as remembering.

—WILLIAM JAMES

"I can't find my glasses."

"They're on your bedside table."

"I looked. They're not there."

"Yes they are. They're on top of the latest issue of *National Geographic,* and your car keys and a dollar in change are there too."

"What do you know, there they are!"

Endless versions of this scenario occur between my wife, Barbara, and me—and I probably don't have to specify which character I am in these exchanges. Each time I am baffled how I could have overlooked the missing object, and equally amazed how my wife can recall small details so perfectly.

Forgetting is a serious concern, because we associate memory loss with mental decline and aging. I admit that each time I can't recall a name, a word, or where my glasses or car keys are hiding, a little fear creeps in. Are these the first warnings of Alzheimer's disease? Have I contracted the second case of mad cow disease in the United States and are these the early signs that my brain is rotting? Should I take more ginkgo?

Here's another typical interchange between Barbara and me:

"Please stop by that new bakery and pick up some fresh bread for dinner."

"Sure. What's the address?"

"You're driving along Grant Street, you pass a pink building on the right, which is across from a parking lot. There's a big pothole shaped like the state of Texas just before you get to the bakery. Can't miss it."

"Thanks, dear. Would that be north or south on Grant?"

"There's a low wall with seven charming aspen trees in front of the bakery."

"Sounds lovely. I'll look up the address myself."

Barbara and I make a good team when we travel. She remembers little details, and I'm there with a map and a compass. I love maps and compasses. I keep maps of most major American cities in a file drawer, from which I select the appropriate one before going on a trip. I also own six compasses, one of which I keep on my desktop. Even now it is faithfully pointing north—a constant in my life, which I find immensely consoling. Even so, I check it several times a day to make sure nothing has changed. If the poles shift, as some doomsayers warn, I want to be among the first to know. Nothing like staying current.

A lot of men share my enthusiasms. While in Paris a few years ago, Barbara and I took the Metro to the Arc de Triomphe. When we surfaced from the subway, we encountered a maze of streets and were disoriented. I brandished my compass and map and within seconds we were no longer confused. Then I glanced to my right and saw another couple, obviously Americans. The man was engaged in his own compass-and-map ritual. The woman was impatient and said to him, "Why not ask?" He and I looked at each other, saw each other's map and compass, and burst out laughing.

My wife's ability to navigate around town without a street map or address may seem unrelated to her ability to locate objects I can't find. But cognitive psychologists say these skills are connected and are related to gender. I am fond of these research findings because they de-pathologize my flawed memory. Instead of a disease, I seem simply to be suffering from a guy thing.

Over the past few decades, numerous studies from many cultures have shown a consistent finding: Men score higher than women on standard tests of spatial abilities such as reading maps, learning mazes, and rotating three-dimensional objects in their imaginations. Even male animals navigate better than their female counterparts.

However, psychologists Irwin Silverman and Marion Eals of York University suggest that these differences are not absolute.[1] Women, they say, excel at different types of spatial skills, and the gender differences may be related to our evolutionary history. In earliest human times, males predominantly hunted and females foraged, which are activities requiring different spatial skills. Hunters needed to be able to maintain their orientation while pursuing game over great distances and over unfamiliar terrain in order to return home. They looked for key landmarks and big topographical features—the overall picture—and kept a rough estimate in their heads of the direction and distance they had traveled. In contrast, women, in order to be successful gatherers, attuned themselves to minute changes in their environment in order to locate, identify, and discriminate edible from inedible roots and plants. A good forager would have developed the ability always to keep an eye out for subtle features in the local environment, even when engaged in other tasks. So it isn't that men had spatial skills and women had none. Their spatial skills differed because they needed to be different.

Silverman and Eals devised tests for their hypothesis. They left subjects alone for two minutes in a small office containing a variety of personal and work-related items. Some subjects were told to memorize the objects and their location in the room (directed learning), while other subjects were asked merely to wait in the room for a few minutes (incidental learning). In both groups, women consistently outscored men on naming objects and specifying their locations. The differences were greatest for incidental learning of the location of objects. Women were able to tune in to the details of their surroundings without really trying to do so and without paying much attention. Men, in contrast, had to be told to pay attention to particulars before they did so.

Psychologist James Dabbs of Georgia State University replicated these findings. "If you make men learn and be interested in the objects in the room, they'll learn well," he says.[2]

Many studies have indicated that men typically navigate in terms of distances and specific directions. Jean Choi, a graduate student in Silverman's laboratory, found that women, in contrast, use specific landmarks and concepts such as right or left turns. She found that women who use landmarks to learn a route perform better than women who use distances and directions, while men perform worse when they use landmarks and better when they rely on distances.[3]

German scientists at Ulm University report similar findings.[4] They used sophisticated computer tests to plot the brain's electrical activity in male and female subjects who were asked to navigate through a maze. They discovered that men used part of their left brain while women used part of their right brain, and that men accomplished the task faster. They confirmed the above research showing that women look for landmarks to orient themselves, while men estimate how far and in what direction they travel.

I have seized on these findings and have twisted them into an excuse for forgetting where I leave my car keys. I tell my wife that I'm concentrating on large-scale, lofty issues—the Big Picture—and can't be bothered with the small stuff. She does not appear to be impressed.

Can Our Memory Be Too Good?

Alan Watts, the Buddhist scholar, proposed the existence of a mental faculty he called forgettory, which is the flip side of memory. There are times, Watts maintained, when we need to forget things, to let them slip away into the unremembered past. We need both abilities, he said, for a healthy mind.

Imagine a world in which everything that happened was remembered. Nothing went unnoticed, nothing was forgotten, and every event could be recalled on command. It would be hell on earth. Privacy would not exist and there would be no place to hide. Our justice system would be revolutionized: We would no longer need multiple witnesses, because the memory of even a single witness would be perfect and would not need corroborating. Even if there were no human witnesses to a crime, gadgets with perfect recall could record things we did not notice, and could serve the function of the expert witness. We are inching toward such a world, and we need to be cautious.

For example, in many industrialized countries, traffic cameras are becoming the norm. In Germany, drivers have been warned to stop making rude gestures at the cameras or they could be charged with insulting the police. A Bavarian court ruled in 2000 that a driver who held up his middle finger while passing a traffic camera was addressing the police officers themselves rather than the equipment, which constituted an offense. The motorist said he didn't think the camera was switched on, but the video footage, with its infallible memory, proved him wrong.[5]

How can a gesture be obscene if no human is present to be offended? In a world drifting toward perfect memory, questions such as this will become more relevant. In such a world, privacy is certain to become increasingly valued, and forgetting more highly prized.

The Curse of a Perfect Memory

In the 1920s, the Russian neuropsychologist Alexander L. Luria began to study S. V. Shereshevski, a Moscow newspaper employee whose remarkable photographic recall came to public attention. In laboratory tests Shereshevski was asked to recall countless lists of formulas, symbols, words, musical scores, and items of nonsense, which he unfailingly did, with his eyes closed and his finger tracing imaginary outlines. Luria discovered that the man was engaging in visualizing the things he was asked to remember, building associations which later aided his recall. Shereshevski also constructed complex associations with a range of feelings and emotions, such as the weight and taste of a word, and how words tickled his hand as he imagined them slipping through his fingers.

These patterns were so rich they sometimes caused confusion. For example, if a familiar person happened to be dressed in clothes Shereshevski had never seen before, or if he or she used new gestures or expressions, this new information would produce sensations that prevented him from recalling the person's name.

Aside from its depth and breadth, one of the most remarkable features of Shereshevski's memory was its longevity. When Luria tested him five, ten, fifteen, and twenty years later, he found that his subject could recall all the information he had ever been given, even adding details such as what Luria had been wearing on the day of the original experiment and what the weather was.

But Shereshevski was also unable to forget, and his mind became crowded by vast quantities of information of no consequence, which normal individuals would not have remembered in the first place. He could not function at an abstract level because his mind was flooded with trivia. Shereshevski became haunted by the contents of his superb memory. Events he would have gladly forgotten clung tenaciously, losing nothing of their emotional vividness over the years.[6,7]

When Doctors Need to Forget

Becoming a doctor is highly dependent on memorization, and students who do not have the gift of a good memory do not survive the premed college years and the rigors of medical school. Because of the emphasis on memorizing, we overlook the fact that physicians often need to forget in order to be competent.

Consider what is required of a doctor when a patient seeks a second opinion from her. The patient presents the medical records to the new physician, asks her to set aside the earlier diagnosis, and render a fresh judgment. If the second physician cannot forget the first doctor's opinion for the moment, she will be influenced by the original diagnosis and may simply echo the first doctor's conclusion. In one study, when doctors were given a diagnostic label for a particular case and were asked to make an independent assessment, they were more likely to reiterate the initial diagnosis than physicians to whom the earlier diagnosis was not disclosed.[8]

A similar situation exists in the courtroom. Judges often ask jurors to disregard inadmissible evidence and pretrial publicity in their deliberations about the guilt or innocence of a defendant. Numerous studies with mock jurors have shown that this is extremely difficult to do. Even in the face of explicit instructions to ignore such information, jurors are more likely to convict than those who were never exposed to this information.[9,10]

Animals Forget Too

Experiments in animals show that forgetting can be dangerously efficient, because it may involve the loss of vital skills such as procuring food. Brighton University researcher Tim Fullford and his colleagues trained an octopus named Roger Moore to unscrew a jam jar containing tasty crabmeat. Roger, who was named after one of the actors who played the James Bond role, took twenty-one minutes to open the jar and retrieve the food on his first attempt, but over the next three days he got his time down to a minute. Although his short-term memory was excellent, when the trainers gave him a break for a day or two he completely forgot how to do it.[11]

The Dark Side of Memory

Addiction researchers have long believed that an addict's desire for drugs such as cocaine is due to the satisfaction of cravings by brain chemicals such as dopamine. Now there is evidence of the opposite situation—that dopamine and other brain chemicals may not only satisfy drug cravings, but stimulate them as well by activating memories of past drug experiences. When researchers stimulated a memory center in the hippocampus region of the brain of rats that had been weaned from cocaine addiction, they found that powerful cravings for cocaine returned, as if an ignition switch had been turned.[12,13] The researchers suspect that merely remembering drug experiences may flip addicts back into addiction, and that the brain's memory center in the hippocampus is involved. This is consistent with the stories addicts tell—that simple reminders of previous drug use, such as passing a particular street corner or bumping into a former addict friend, may trigger drug-seeking behavior.

Rewriting Our Script

Most people say they deplore false memories and that they always want to remember things the way they really were. Healthcare professionals also generally ask their patients to face their situation honestly. But false memories, distortions, and illusions of the past can promote health, even when they are flat-out wrong. In one research study of women with breast cancer, those who responded to their initial diagnosis with brazen denial had almost the same survival statistics over a ten-year period as those who faced their diagnoses with openness and honesty.[14]

UCLA social psychologist Shelley E. Taylor has discovered that almost anyone will adopt a coping strategy based on illusion if life becomes harsh enough. She says, "[R]epression and denial increase in magnitude as the threatening content of information increases."[15]

Taylor continues, "Traditional concepts of mental health promote the idea that an accurate or correct view of the self is critical to the healthy self-concept. But decades of empirical research suggest that a quite different conclusion is merited. Increasingly, we must view the psychologically healthy person not as someone who sees things as they are but as someone who sees things as he or she would like them to be. Effective functioning in everyday life appears to depend upon interrelated positive illusions, systematic small distortions of reality that make things appear better than they are."[16]

But creating an effective illusion is a delicate matter. The illusion must not be so out of line with reality that it is easily disconfirmed or falsified by others. That's why, Taylor says, the illusions people employ are usually mild, not extreme—they must be able to slip by without being challenged by one's friends and acquaintances.[17]

Spinning the Past

Dieter Frey, a Munich psychologist, has shown that trauma patients can dramatically affect health outcomes by how they interpret past events. He interviewed three hundred accident victims at the University Clinic in Kiel and followed their clinical course. His subjects had been injured at work, playing sports, or driving, and their injuries ranged from broken bones to concussion. Two days following admission, Frey asked them whose fault the accident had been, and whether the patients believed it could have been avoided, and if they felt they could influence their recovery. Patients who said that the accident was not their fault, they could not have avoided it, and they had learned something useful from the experience, were discharged in approximately twenty days. They suffered fewer major complications such as blood clots and heart problems. But those who believed they could have prevented the accident or asked questions such as "Why me?" required an average of forty days to recover and stayed off work an extra two months compared to the other group.[18]

"With these results we can predict, two days after an accident, how quickly a patient will recover," Frey comments. He urges doctors and nurses to get patients involved in healing themselves: "If they do that right, they will have, in effect, a free therapy at hand." Should we help people construct the past in ways that foster recovery, even though this may be at variance with the facts? Which is more important: helping trauma victims remember things accurately, or helping them remember in a way that promotes a better clinical course?

Emphasizing positive events in our past and ignoring others can be a healthy mental strategy. This is particularly dramatic in athletes.[19] Take the case of the French professional golfer Jean Van de Velde. In July 1999, Van de Velde, who was almost unknown, riveted the golf world by leading the British Open in the last phase of the tournament. Going into the final hole, he held an impressive three-shot lead and seemed assured of victory. Then one of the most stunning meltdowns in the history of professional golf occurred. Van de Velde landed wild shots in the rough and the water, finishing with a triple-bogey and a three-way tie for the lead, which he also lost, as millions of golf fans watched from around the world.

The London sports pages the next day predicted that Van de Velde would be haunted the rest of his life by the memory of the disaster. But although he was shaken initially, he did not agonize about what might have been. He explained the rationale for some of his decisions, although they backfired, and he philosophized that golf is only a game and just a single aspect of his life. Van de Velde was happy to have been the focus of international fame, if only briefly, but added, "I don't live in the past."[20]

In contrast, consider the experience of Donnie Moore, a pitcher for the California Angels baseball team. In early October 1986, the Angels were nearing victory over the Boston Red Sox in the American League Championship series. It was the ninth inning of the fifth game in the series, which they led by a score of 5 to 2. The Angels needed only this victory to clinch the series and go on to the World Series. When the Red Sox narrowed the lead to 5 to 4, the Angels brought in their ace relief pitcher Donnie Moore to face Red Sox hitter Dave Henderson. Moore threw two quick strikes, then Henderson feebly fouled off the next pitch, obviously overpowered by Moore.

Then, against the odds, Henderson slammed Moore's next pitch for a game-winning home run. The Angels players and their fans looked on in disbelief. They failed to recover, and Boston progressed to the World Series.

The team and their fans bounced back, but Donnie Moore didn't. Henderson's home run haunted him. In spite of encouragement from his teammates, who pointed out the many games he had saved, Moore could only focus on the one fateful pitch. The media constantly harped on the disastrous incident and refused to let it die. Moore descended into deep depression, and his career and marriage were soon on the rocks. His situation ended violently. As an Associated Press release described on July 19, 1989, "Tormented by the memory of one pitch, and despondent over his failing career and marital troubles, former California Angels pitcher Donnie Moore shot his wife numerous times before killing himself, police said." Dave Pinter, Moore's agent, observed, "Even when he was told that one pitch doesn't make a season, he couldn't get over it. That home run killed him."

Jean Van de Velde was able to use selective forgetting to build what psychologists call a positive "self-schema."[21] Donnie Moore could not, and it cost his wife and him their lives.

The inability to forget personal failings is an ancient human problem that, like most of the great challenges we face, resonates in mythology. In his book *Achilles in Vietnam*, psychiatrist Jonathan Shay describes similarities between the trauma of combat in Vietnam and in Homer's *The Iliad*. In an incident in *The Iliad*, Achilles becomes overwhelmed with grief because he failed to cover for a comrade who was slain. He feels "pierced by memory"—like thousands of returning veterans of the wars of our time.[22]

Purposeful Forgetting

Most of us assume that we can't reconstruct our memories at will. If we try to forget something and replace it with a different thought, the rejected memory only becomes more vivid. As a French proverb says,

"To want to forget something is to think of it."[23] And as *Alice in Wonderland* author Lewis Carroll noted, "Again and again I have said to myself, on lying down at night, after a day embittered by some vexatious matter, 'I will not think of it any more! . . . It can do no good whatever to go through it again. I will think of something else!' And in another ten minutes I have found myself, once more, in the very thick of the miserable business, and torturing myself, to no purpose, with all the old troubles."[24]

Recent experiments, however, suggest that we may be able to willfully forget under certain circumstances. Researchers have shown that if people practice avoiding the memory of certain words, they become more successful at forgetting them when they are later asked to recall them. This may have practical importance. For instance, evidence suggests that children who have been sexually abused by a trusted caregiver forget that experience far more frequently than do kids abused by a stranger.[25] Researchers suggest that abused children use indirect reminders, such as the presence of the abuser, as cues to avoid thinking about the actual abuse.[26]

Other investigators, however, suggest that trying to forget unwanted thoughts may backfire, assuring the very state of mind one had hoped to avoid.[27]

Preventing Age-Related Memory Loss

Memory loss is not inevitable with aging. Staying mentally and physically active are the main preventives, says a report from the Institute for the Study of Aging (ISOA) and the International Longevity Center-USA (ILC-USA), "Achieving and Maintaining Cognitive Vitality with Aging."[28,29] "People who think there's a pill that is going to keep the mind in top form are mistaken," says Robert N. Butler, MD, president of ILC-USA and former director of the National Institute on Aging. "But the good news is that most people can keep their mental capacities from declining just by doing simple things like walking, reading the newspaper, taking a music class, and getting help for problems like stress and depression." Instead of telling older patients to take it easy, Butler says, "They [physicians] should recommend active, positive uses of one's head and not accept losses. Just remind [them], use it or lose it."

To prevent or limit cognitive decline, the cognitive vitality report makes seven recommendations:

- *Lifelong learning.* This includes the intellectual stimulation that comes from doing memory exercises and playing intellectually stimulating games.
- *Exercise.* This increases blood supply and oxygen to the brain. Even moderate activities such as walking help.
- *Daily activities.* Older people should consider remaining active in the workforce, traveling, volunteering, gardening, and joining social events.
- *Stress reduction.* Meditation, muscle relaxation training, and yoga can be helpful.
- *Sleep.* Sleep disorders are common in older people; decrease in rapid eye movement or dream sleep can interfere with cognitive function.
- *Emotional stability.* Depression is particularly common in white men, and, if protracted, should be dealt with by medical professionals.
- *Nutrition.* A balanced diet is more important for older people than the currently popular "anti-aging" drugs and nutritional fads. Although the report concedes that estrogen and antioxidants may potentially preserve cognitive vitality, it stipulates that the findings are preliminary and that the risks of supplements such as melatonin, dehydroepiandrosterone (DHEA), and human growth hormone outweigh the touted benefits.

Gene Manipulation

Recently, a team of Princeton neurobiologists identified a gene that is connected with memory retention in experiments with mice, and by manipulating the gene they were able to stimulate better memory during learning tasks.[30] The scientists suggested that it might be possible to modify genes in mammals to enhance memory and intelligence, just like in the mice. Some experts, however, such as neuroscientist Tim Tully of New York's Cold Spring Harbor Laboratory, are concerned about the ethics of using memory-enhancing drugs and gene manipulation to stimulate memory.[31] He suggests that the military would be among the first to use such drugs in soldiers to help them carry out orders with perfect precision. Tully, a pacifist, says, "I would hate to see this understanding perfected for the art of war, for all the covert and overt atrocities that humans push over on each other."

Some parents, wishing to give their progeny every advantage to excel, would also demand the memory-enhancing drugs, just like thousands of parents who wanted human growth hormone (HGH) to make their children grow taller, when this substance became commercially available. Should parents be giving their kids a memory-enhancing pill every morning before they are packed off to school? Could their developing brains handle the increase in information? Would we be creating little Shereshevskis who will sink under the weight of remembered trivia later in life? Will we then need to engineer a "forgetting pill" to help balance things out? Would kids whose parents cannot afford the new memory drugs be disadvantaged and left behind? Would students buy memory enhancers off the street when it is time to cram for exams, and would a new black market spring up?

Mind-Body and Spiritual Approaches to Better Memory

Amid the flurry of interest in herbal, nutritional, and genetic approaches, it is easy to overlook methods such as religious devotion, meditation, yoga, tai chi, and prayer, which have been recognized since antiquity to aid mental clarity and cognitive function.

Spiritual and religious disciplines have been associated with a lower incidence of many major illnesses such as heart disease and cancer.[32,33]

Let us bear in mind, however, that the main purpose of spiritual practice is not to prevent or cure memory loss or anything else, but to connect us with something greater than the individual self—the Absolute, the Divine, or however named. If we forget this, spiritual practices can degenerate to become merely the latest trick in our medical tool kit.

Is Forgetting Good?

Nature has endowed us with the capacity both to remember and to forget. This dual system has survived throughout our long evolutionary history, presumably because it serves a valuable function. Is it wise to unbalance it merely because we can? This is not an easy question to answer, because almost everyone would prefer a better memory to the one they have. One way of approaching the issue is to see how forgetting operates in people with terrific memories. If forgetting plays a prominent role in their lives, perhaps we should be more tolerant of it in our own.

Tatiana Cooley, a twenty-seven-year-old administrative assistant, was the 1999 winner of the National Memory Champion contest.[34] The participants were challenged to memorize lengthy poems, thousands of words and numbers, pages of names and faces, and rearranged decks of cards. Cooley did not pop memory-enhancing pills and had not had her genes manipulated. She won the old-fashioned way—relying on classic association techniques dating to the Greeks, which rely on building visual images and stories linking incoming information to what she already knew. You might expect her memory to be near-perfect, like Shereshevski's, but Cooley considers herself horribly forgetful. "I live by Post-Its," she revealed. "I'm incredibly absent-minded."

Is there a lesson here? If forgetting is a trait of someone with a world-class memory, should we be so eager to exterminate it with gene tricks and miracle pills?[35]

Memory Prostheses

One of my favorite Web sites is Word Spy, which keeps track of recently coined words and phrases (www.wordspy.com). One such term is "memory prosthesis," defined as a device that helps or enables a person to remember things.

People have been searching for suitable memory prostheses for a long time. When Napoleon went to war two centuries ago, he used a traveling filing cabinet as a memory aid and as a way to keep abreast of the things he needed to know.[36] It was the most advanced form of information retrieval ever used in warfare up to that time—so advanced that the methodical Duke of Wellington, his nemesis, never hit upon it.

The amount of information Napoleon had to process pales in comparison with the data which washes over us every day. Our memories simply can't handle the load. A friend called me twice this week and left a message on my answering machine. I returned both calls and each time he confessed, "Gee, I really can't remember why I called." This is the sort of thing that causes us to doubt our faculties and reach for the ginkgo—if we can remember where we put the bottle.

But perhaps we are too harsh on ourselves. We are required to remember more things than ever before—which means that we have more opportunities for forgetting. This magnifies our sense of forgetfulness. This would not be a problem if we could keep remembering and forgetting in perspective, but we can't. We blame ourselves for what we forget, but we don't credit ourselves with the fantastic quantity of information we process and recall each day of our lives. If we actually tallied the things we remember in a day's time against the things that slip by, we might conclude that our memories are far better than we assume they are.

There is a danger of being sucked into a negative feedback loop where forgetting is concerned. Our fear of forgetting can lead to hypervigilance about how our memory is performing, so that successive forgetfulness becomes increasingly obvious. Eventually, we begin to pathologize our cognitive life, and the resulting anxiety and worry can make us even more forgetful.

We are drowning in reminders of the fallibility of our memory. Many of our daily activities are little more than a hedge against forgetting, constantly reminding us that our memory can't be trusted. The alarm in the morning is a don't-forget-to-wake-up device. The preprogrammed, automatic coffeemaker is a memoryproof gadget to get us up and going. The daily schedules we tattoo into our prosthetic Palm Pilots and laptops are digital warnings to prevent our forgetting where we should be and what we should be doing. Our computers are programmed with the assumption that we have a faulty memory. Mine repeatedly asks questions that emphasize my incompetence, such as "Did you remember to back up your files today?" Screensavers are available with the message, "DON'T FORGET TO BREATHE!"

Then there are all those PINs and passwords to Web sites, telephones, ATMs, and e-mail, which we all forget. Not to worry. Just yesterday I bumped into a Web site through which you can retrieve your forgotten password. I'd share the name of the site with you, but I forgot it. We are sinking into an infinite regression of reminders, from the tinny alarms on our watches to the irritating bleeps on the microwave oven.

Is a truce possible in the war on forgetting?

Instead of combating forgetfulness head-on, I'm trying to make peace with it. I find that I can increasingly find a silver lining in my recall failures. Consequently, instead of beating up on myself, I've even begun to feel slightly proud of being an excellent forgetter.

For example, in the process of becoming a physician, I was cranked out of a premed and medical school program that rewarded memorization. But there was a dirty little secret: The medical school faculty knew all along that the brains of even the best students were sieves, and that we'd hang on to only a fraction of the things they required us to commit to memory. Moreover, they knew some of the stuff they crammed into us was flat-out wrong and should be forgotten. As one prof admitted, "In five years, you'll realize that half the things we're teaching you are correct, and half are wrong. Unfortunately, we can't tell one half from the other." So it was a good thing that I forgot much of what I learned in medical school. Forgetting cleans out the attic and makes room for new and better information.

George Savile, first Marquess of Halifax (1633–1695), said, "Some men's memory is like a box, where a man should mingle his jewels with his old shoes."[37] But the size of the box is limited. Do we really want to hang on to the smelly old shoes? These days I'm getting more comfortable with cleaning out the box. I'm going for the jewels instead of the shoes, and I'm praying for the wisdom to tell them apart.

3

Novelty

*The real voyage of discovery consists not in seeking new
landscapes but in having new eyes.*

—MARCEL PROUST

One morning around 1820, Gustav Fechner, a young professor of physics in Leipzig, awoke, it is said, with a realization that prompted him to shout, "Eureka!" Fechner had suddenly become aware of what would come to be called the Psychophysical Law, an enormously general principle that helps explain why a sense of novelty fizzles out with repeated exposure to the same experience, and why even pleasurable events eventually become boring.

Fechner realized that in order to experience something over and over again at the original level of intensity, we have to keep jacking up the energy level of the stimulus each time the event is repeated. Examples are commonplace in everyone's life. For instance, my first computer seemed magical to me, even though it was undeniably primitive and slow as molasses. But at the time I was blissfully unaware of these shortcomings, and the machine seemed to glow with a celestial halo, whose radiance spread throughout my life as it transformed one mundane task after another. With time, however, the novelty faded and the magic wore off. Like an addict, I needed an additional stimulus to rekindle the old excitement. Along with all the other cyberjunkies I know, I embarked on a never-ending series of updates and expansions, replacing one machine after another. Yet these incremental improvements never replicated the frisson I had experienced on taking the leap from having no computer at all, to using my first, clunky machine.

I didn't know it at the time, but I was in the thrall of Fechner's Psychophysical Law. I was a human version of a three-way light bulb, whose levels of brightness are keyed to 40, 80, and 120 watts. When you turn on such a bulb in a dark room, you experience a sudden increase in brightness as you go from complete darkness to the 40-watt level. Turn the switch a second time, and although you double the electrical energy from 40 to 80 watts, your actual sensation of brightness is not commensurate with a doubling. And when you turn the switch a third time, boosting the bulb's energy to 120 watts, the increased brightness is hardly noticeable.

My computer experience paralleled this situation to a tee. My most profound experiential surge was in the transition from being computerless to using a computer for the first time—turning the light bulb on in the dark. The technological add-ons—increasing the brightness, so to speak—never duplicated this experience; indeed, each succeeding update seemed to contribute less and less to my computer joy.

Kids get involved in a similar process with video games. The elation they experience from a new game fades quickly, and they require increasing jolts of sensory input in the form of newer, fancier, and usually more expensive amusements—a runaway scenario that the video game marketers exploit with precision, to the chagrin of parents.

Almost any behavior that depends on electronic gadgets follows this pattern. A prime example is physical fitness programs. Millions of individuals have come to equate exercise with computerized treadmills, stair steps, bicycles, rowing machines, and so on. These machines hold one's attention initially, but their attraction eventually dwindles for most users. The equipment seldom wears out; it is merely replaced by fancier gadgets that promise to deliver more fitness with less effort. The new machines typically wind up gathering dust in garages and attics, or as derelicts in stores that have sprouted all over the country that resell secondhand exercise equipment.

The ultimate electronic gadgets are antifitness machines. They belong to the military and are designed to break things. All our computerized planes, ships, tanks, bombs, and missiles, like our personal computers and exercise equipment, eventually lose their allure and are replaced periodically—sometimes, it seems, for no good reason. The rationale, of course, always hinges on national security; the new weapons systems, we hear, are more modern and sophisticated and will make us safer. The impression of many, however, is that the new weaponry is chosen for reasons that have less to do with national security than with other factors—including the fact that increasingly powerful stimuli are required to generate the same level of excitement, whether in the domain of toys, cars, or the tools of war.

The Psychophysical Law is particularly applicable to authors. For most writers the greatest thrill of their career is the publication of their first book, and many authors spend the rest of their professional lives trying to recapture that experience. This task usually proves elusive, causing many writers to experience a perpetual sense of inadequacy, of coming up short.

Fechner's Law also helps explains certain publishing patterns. A classic example is diet books, which are published in an unending stream and which always occupy, it seems, a slot or two on the bestseller lists. Almost any new dietary program can capture one's attention initially and may even be effective. But the new plan eventually becomes boring and is abandoned, making way for a newer, novel program—a more powerful stimulus—and the next chartbuster.

The thing that is so special about the Psychophysical Law is its broad range of applications. Neuroscientist Bernard J. Baars, of San Diego's Neurosciences Institute, is a fan of Fechner's insight, and he describes how it applies to all the senses as well as to such perceptions as heat, pain, and muscular effort. The Psychophysical Law explains, says Baars, "why the first bite of chocolate cake tastes so good, the second less so, and [the] third much less; that what causes a fashion sensation this year is gone the next; and why as we get older, days and weeks that once seemed to last forever begin to flash by faster and faster. It may explain why millionaires need to earn more money the richer they become, and why addicts may need higher drug doses over time. In all these examples, equal increments in objective quantities appear smaller and smaller against a growing basis of comparison; and comparison is the essence of the Psychophysical Law. It is a classic piece of scientific discovery, an elegant, precise, general and fully predictable feature of conscious sensation."[1]

Fechner's law seems so obvious, so ordinary, that one may wonder why it should be considered a breakthrough at all. The fact is I have painted a simplified picture of the Psychophysical Law. The souped-up version is a little more elegant. It says that equal increases in the energy of a sensory input are experienced as smaller and smaller increments of subjective intensity; or, to state it in reverse, equal or arithmetic increases in the intensity of a subjective experience require geometric increases in the physical energy contained in the sensory stimulus. Over the years, Fechner's original insight was refined by E. H. Weber and others to what is sometimes called the Weber-Fechner Law, which states that the magnitude of a subjective sensation increases proportional to the logarithm of the stimulus intensity.[2,3]

It is somewhat surprising that Fechner (1801–1887), in his nineteenth year, would come up with a law dealing with sensory experiences, because sensation and perception don't usually concern physicists, and he was a gifted physicist. Fechner was not a typical, classical physicist, however, but a brilliant, enigmatic individual who was passionately concerned with the operation of the mind. For example, he developed a philosophy that all matter possessed consciousness to some degree. At one point in his life, he stared at the sun as an experiment and damaged his retinas, which prompted him to wear bandages over his eyes for three years in a futile attempt to regain his vision. Some said Fechner was mad; others heralded him as a genius who saw deeply into the realms of consciousness.

Staying Fresh

Some premodern cultures understood the importance of novelty in craftwork. It has been said of Native American women that their baskets were their poems, the shaping of them their sculpture, and that they wove into them the story of their lives and loves. Especially prized were baskets made by women of the Mescalero Apache tribe in the desert of New Mexico. The rich variety of their creations was almost guaranteed, because tradition decreed that no two baskets could be ornamented identically. This meant that the elaboration of new designs was continually unfolding. When two baskets were discovered to be identical, as occasionally happened by accident, the weaver was subjected to grave consequences that were decided by a council of her peers. Sometimes it was decided that the offending basket might be changed, but if not it was destroyed. But the full extent of punishment for this serious transgression was known only to insiders and was a secret part of Mescalero tradition.[4]

Buckminster Fuller, the celebrated philosopher, inventor, and designer who gave the world the geodesic dome, understood the importance of novelty. During the 1960s and 1970s, "Bucky" was lionized by a generation of young thinkers who were irreverently pushing the boundaries in both the arts and the sciences. He advised people to change their occupation every ten years, even though they might be highly successful at what they were already doing. Only by changing channels periodically could one prevent boredom and stagnation, he maintained, and ensure continuing creativity and fulfillment.

On the surface, Fuller's advice sounds reckless. It often takes a decade or longer to achieve success in one's career. Why bail out, especially if things are going well? It all comes down to that chocolate cake. The second bite is always less satisfying than the first. Eventually all bites become nearly tasteless, and all one gets is the calories.

Meditation

One of the time-honored ways of preserving the freshness of experience is through meditation.

In a classic experiment during the 1960s, physician-researchers Akira Kasamatsu and Tomio Hirai of the University of Tokyo, tracked the brain waves of Zen Buddhist teachers and their best students while they were repeatedly exposed to the same high-pitched sound while meditating, and they compared these responses to those of control subjects with no meditation experience. The controls gradually became habituated to the stimuli; eventually their brain waves ceased to register when a sound was made. In contrast, the Zen meditators did not become habituated. Their brain waves continued to respond to the stimuli, as if they were hearing each sound afresh for the first time.[5]

One of the goals of meditation is to stay in the moment and attend fully to every experience that comes along. Each thought and sensation is allowed to stand on its own without censorship or comparison. Meditators who master this skill discover that the present is continually renewed and novelty is preserved, as if one is being born anew in every moment.

But the thirst for novelty can be pathological. If we crave titillation, we cannot rest in the present but are constantly looking to the future for ways of relieving the emptiness we feel. Eventually, we may realize we are on the wrong track and that we need to focus on the fullness of the present. If we do so, we, like the meditators, may discover something extraordinary—that repetitious, ordinary experiences can be transformed into novel, fresh perceptions. This paradox ranks as one of the most profound realizations of our capabilities as humans.

Armed with this insight, we are equipped to challenge Bucky's recommendation that we change our occupation once every decade in order to preserve a sense of newness and creativity. Instead of changing our job, we can change our response *to* it. If we do so, going to work every day can be as novel an experience as hearing each sound as if for the first time is for the meditators—and who, we can presume, experience that third bite of chocolate cake as vividly as the first.

This reference to eating is more than metaphor. The ability to be in the present dramatically affects our response to food. Author and nutritionist Debra Kesten is convinced that a major reason underlying the epidemic of obesity in America is that we have forgotten how to attend, to pay attention, to the simple act of eating. In her admirable books *Feeding the Body, Nourishing the Soul* and *The Healing Secrets of Food,* she describes how we are no longer present during a meal.[6,7] We are detached, spaced out, split off, and essentially absent from the cere- mony of mealtime, simultaneously watching television, surfing the Web, reading, doing homework, talking on cell phones, or driving, all the while patting ourselves on the back for our ability to engage in that modern curse, multitasking. This mindless way of eating may expand our productivity, but it also expands our waistlines. When we eat mindlessly, nothing satisfies, so we eat more. It isn't just that the third bite of chocolate cake is unsatisfying; the first bite is, too, because we are so minimally aware of what we are putting into our mouths. We might as well be eating cardboard—which, unfortu- nately, is what much of our diet has come to resemble.

Thus Kesten concludes that diet programs don't work well unless we learn to be fully present when we eat. Genuinely focusing on our food results in an increase in the pleasure we derive from it, which means we eat less. The bottom line is that we need more than fresh food; we need a fresh *experience* of food.

Kesten stresses the spirituality of eating, which is about more than quickly saying grace and then diving in. Eating spiritually involves thankfulness that we do not go to bed hungry; a reverence for the plants and animals that nourish us; a sense of connectedness with all of life; and gratitude to those whose labor provides our food.

In his superb book *In Praise of Slowness,* author Carl Honoré describes how we can slow down and relax into saner ways of order- ing our lives on many levels, including eating. If we are willing to do so, it is possible to escape the tyranny of fast food, fast eating, and the burdens of obesity with which so many people struggle.[8] Each meal can be a new meal, each bite a new bite, and the pleasures that result can substitute for the calories.

Neophobia

Neophobia is the fear of new things, and neophobes are individuals who cringe from novelty in favor of predictability, repetition, and routine.

Neophobia is widespread in the animal world and has been studied in rats by researchers Sonia Cavigelli and Martha McClintock at the University of Chicago.[9] They selected two types of rats from pairs of brothers—those who were brave when confronted with novel situations, and those who were scared when faced with new challenges. The researchers found two main differences in the groups following a new experience. First, the fearful animals had a blood level of the stress hormone corticosterone 20 percent higher than their brave brothers. Second, there was a major difference in longevity. The median lifespan for the neophobes was 599 days, while the median survival time for the fearless rats was 701 days—a 17 percent difference.

The researchers aren't sure whether these findings can be extended to humans, but my hunch is that there are areas in which they indeed apply. I have always been struck by the capacity of widows to adapt to the deaths of their husbands—to pick up and carry on by accepting changes and new challenges—neophilia, as it were. In comparison, men seem almost neophobic when their spouses die, much less capable of making the transition to new circumstances.

If the above study with rats is any guide, the difficulty men experience in handling new situations may cause surges in stress hormones and an increase in stress-related illnesses. The differences in how they respond to new situations may help explain why, on average, American women live around seven years longer than men.

Neophobia may also help explain the high death rates in men following retirement. When faced with a new situation—no job to go to every day, the necessity of finding new friends and alternative ways of staying occupied—many men despair. This variety of neophobia may help explain why, for many men, job retirement is hugely stressful and too often a death sentence.

There are times, however, when it is good to avoid new situations. Particularly in dangerous or threatening environments, it may be wisest to play it safe and stick with the familiar. Just because an experience is new doesn't mean it's safe or healthy. As in most situations, the key is balance—hitting the right note between the old and the new, between neophobia and neophilia.

We physicians are faced with the challenges of novelty every day. There is an old saying, "Never be the first nor the last doctor to adopt a new therapy." Jumping on the bandwagon of a new treatment can be disastrous if it has not been properly evaluated; so, too, can the avoidance of a new therapy after its benefits have been thoroughly documented.

Neophobia and CAM

Can neophobia help explain how people respond to complementary/alternative medicine (CAM)? Are CAM critics generally more neophobic, less tolerant of novelty and new ideas than CAM proponents? Are patients who choose CAM more like those brave rats than the fearful ones?

Consider, for example, how people respond to the idea of distant healing, which is supported by various controlled studies of healing intentions and intercessory prayer in both human and nonhuman biological systems.[10,11,12] Many individuals feel threatened when they confront this empirical evidence for the first time. Sometimes this response borders on terror. French scientist Jean-Bernard-Léon Foucault (1819–1868), famous for the pendulum that bears his name, was refreshingly honest about the horror he experienced when confronted with the possibility that human consciousness might act remotely in the world. He said, "If I saw a straw moved by the action of my will, I should be terrified. . . . If the influence of mind upon matter does not cease at the surface of the skin, there is no safety left in the world for anyone."[13] Foucault's contemporary, Hermann von Helmholtz (1821–1894), generally regarded as one of the outstanding physicists of the nineteenth century, agreed, saying, "I cannot believe it. Neither the testimony of all the Fellows of the Royal Society, nor even the evidence of my own senses would lead me to believe in the transmission of thought from one person to another independently of the recognized channels of sensation. It is clearly impossible."[14] Responses such as these persist to this day. Recently, a well-known scientist, rejecting a scientific paper for publication that dealt with the distant manifestations of consciousness, exclaimed, "This is the sort of thing I would not believe, even if it really happened."[15]

These responses express undiluted prejudice, and it would be good if they were dulled. Fortunately, this indeed seems to happen, just as the Psychophysical Law predicts. With repeated exposure to ideas that are initially experienced as outrageous, the threat posed by these concepts is often perceived less vividly. As this process unfolds, even die-hard skeptics such as Foucault and von Helmholtz can become more tolerant and open to the evidence supporting the new possibilities. One's initial confrontation with a challenging idea like distant healing may be experienced as offensive; with repeated exposure to the idea, however, one can get used to the possibility. Fanatical, knee-jerk criticism abates. The critics' claws gradually retract and the evidence is given a fair hearing. It is not unusual to hear skeptics eventually claim, "I thought of it first!"[16]

The Pleasures of Prejudice

Many radical ideas throughout history have benefited from Fechner's great principle. Consider the notion that freedom is an inalienable right of all humans. Many of the redeeming social movements of the past two centuries are derived from this audacious concept: the abolition of slavery, child labor laws, women's rights, universal suffrage, racial and gender equality, and the freedom of religious expression. All these began as radical, fringe movements that the larger society initially condemned, often violently; but even the political parties that initially opposed them now generally champion all these developments as inherently valid.

The Psychophysical Law can help us understand how such shifts in attitude happen, even in people who hate freedom. There is a distinct pleasure that is experienced by bigots and haters, which is obvious to anyone who has known such an individual up-close. Such persons *enjoy* their prejudices; they derive satisfaction and delight from them. The Psychophysical Law predicts that these pleasures, like any pleasant sensation, can be worn down and attenuated. Thus haters such as Nazi skinheads are typically most vehement in their youth, but often mellow as they age. The Psychophysical Law also dictates that if the pleasures of prejudice are to be maintained at a certain level, the stimulus underlying the perception must be increased in intensity. Perhaps this is why despots such as Hitler, Stalin, Idi Amin, and Pol Pot continually enlarged the scale of their atrocities throughout their lives.

Wandering, Wondering, and Alzheimer's Disease

Wandering—going about without a fixed destination—helps define us as a species. As mathematician and philosopher Alfred North Whitehead said, "One main factor in the upward trend of animal life has been the power of wandering."[17] The origin of "wander" is related to "wind"—air in motion—and when we humans experience the itch to wander and explore what lies beyond the horizon, we are as unstoppable as the wind.

We wander because we crave novelty and the unfamiliar. This need seems to be basic, like our drive for food, water, or sex.

Wondering, like wandering, is a way of encountering novelty in the form of ideas.

Alzheimer's disease has become commonplace in our society. There is evidence that novelty is one of the most potent ways of preventing Alzheimer's. Studies show that exercise such as walking, which is how we wander, significantly reduces the incidence of Alzheimer's. And wondering, through reading books or doing crossword puzzles, also prevents Alzheimer's. Any mental activity "that will push people to encounter something that isn't routine," said one researcher, can help prevent mental decline. When wandering and wondering are combined, they are more potent than when either is used alone.[18]

Will we ever run out of novelty? Some say we already have. The Bible gave a particularly dismal outlook in Ecclesiastes 1:9 with the observation, "There is no new thing under the sun." But we should not worry. As Ambrose Bierce rejoined in *The Devil's Dictionary*, "There is nothing new under the sun, but there are lots of old things we don't know."[19]

4

Tears

Most men cry better than they speak.
—HENRY DAVID THOREAU

I am fascinated by tears and crying, and the reason may be that I'm an identical twin. By all reports, my brother and I put up quite a fuss as babies. We were both needy—two-pound newborns, two months premature, born on an isolated farm in central Texas, with no incubator or nursery within miles. Our parents and grandparents rallied magnificently and brought us through against great odds. While on the obstetrics service, during medical school, I calculated the statistical likelihood of our survival by weighing a host of factors— twin birth, low birth weight, prematurity, home birth, the absence of hospital support, the pre-antibiotic era, on and on. The odds against our survival turned out to be around a hundred to one. My brother and I have carried a great deal of gratitude through life for the plain fact of having survived a rough beginning.

I've wondered if I outcried my brother or vice versa. It was probably a genuine contest. Studies in a variety of animals show that littermates, including humans, will engage in crying and begging behaviors to attract their parents' attention in order to get more food—what ethologists call "care-soliciting signals." This behavior can backfire in nature, however, because it can attract predators. For example, baby birds whose parents nest in the open or on the ground perform relatively inconspicuous attention-getting displays, while those who nest in safer places such as trees produce louder calls.[1] Since my brother and I had a safe nest and didn't have to worry about predators, we probably screamed our lungs out.

In addition to attracting predators, crying has other downsides. It takes a physical toll on the young by consuming lots of energy, and it doesn't always succeed in attracting more parental attention. Experiments in three species of primates—macaques, vervets, and humans—show that parents tend to play favorites by devoting more attention to the healthier offspring. In some studies, the more the unhealthier offspring cried, the less the mother responded to it. In her study of maternal investment in human twins, psychologist Janet Mann of Georgetown University found that when one twin is healthy and the other sick, the unhealthy twin has to cry longer for maternal attention and feeding than its sibling.[2]

Crying It Out

This brings up the eternal question of whether parents can spoil a crying infant by over-responding to its crying, and whether or not a "cry-it-out" approach is best—leaving babies in their cribs without picking them up, letting them scream until they stop on their own.

The cry-it-out question does not arise when a baby sleeps close to its mother, a practice known as co-sleeping. According to parenting expert Aletha Solter,[3] founder of the Aware Parenting Institute and author of *The Aware Baby* and *Tears and Tantrums*, there is sufficient anthropological evidence to assume that in prehistoric times babies slept on their mothers' bodies or very near. This almost certainly meant that babies were not ignored in favor of crying it out. Co-sleeping is still the norm in many tribal societies around the world.

Why did Western cultures abandon the practice? Solter believes the shift began to take place during the thirteenth century, when Catholic priests started suggesting that mothers not sleep with their infants. The stated reason was the risk of physically smothering the baby. Smothering indeed occurred, but the usual cause was probably inebriated parents, which no doubt evoked intense disapproval from many priests. But the primary reason priests opposed co-sleeping, Solter suggests, was perhaps unconscious and was related to the rise of patriarchy and the fear of too much feminine influence on infants, particularly male children.

The concept of "spoiling" crying infants took hold in industrialized countries during the 1700s. If mothers responded to their cries and held them too much, they might create demanding little monsters. If a home was big enough, parents were encouraged to move the child to a separate sleeping room, which encouraged a cry-it-out strategy. The decline in breastfeeding in the nineteenth century and the rise of bottle-feeding from birth onward were additional factors that helped foster a detached approach to childrearing.

Eventually the cry-it-out perspective began to be trumpeted by psychologists and physicians. John B. Watson, the founder of behaviorism, was hugely influential in childrearing practices in the late nineteenth and early twentieth century. He preferred babies' tears to "too much mother love," which in his writings is almost equated with evil. Too much coddling in childhood reduced the ability of men to "conquer the world," he claimed. "Mothers don't know when they kiss their children and pick them up and rock them, caress them and jiggle them upon their knee, that they are slowly building up a human being totally unable to cope with the world it must later live in." A better approach was to "treat [children] as though they were adults. Let your behavior always be objective and kindly firm. Never hug and kiss them, never let them sit in your lap. If you must, kiss them once on the forehead when they say good night. Shake hands with them in the morning."[4] Equally stern was parenting guru Dr. Luther Emmet Holt, an attending physician to New York Babies Hospital. His book

The Care and Feeding of Children went through thirteen editions between 1894 and 1929, making him the Dr. Spock of his day. Like Watson, he recommended that mothers never sleep with, kiss, or play with their babies, particularly if they are under six months old. If an infant cries for indulgence, it "should simply be allowed to cry it out."[5] Dr. Benjamin Spock, America's parenting sage in the second half of the twentieth century, continued to recommend a cry-it-out approach in his immensely popular *Baby and Child Care.*[6]

Since the 1960s, says Solter, there has been a healthy trend in the opposite direction through what is known as attachment parenting, which is the exact opposite of the cry-it-out approach. Attachment parenting regards infants as vulnerable, feeling humans who need prompt responsiveness and nurturing. Attachment advocates maintain that it is impossible to spoil babies by responding to their cries. Prompt responsiveness, they say, creates a solid foundation of trust and security in infants by one year of age. If parents fail to be responsive, babies typically become clingy and demanding.

Crying it out may be unhealthy physically. Researchers have discovered that even brief separation from the mother results in sharp rises of cortisol in the infant, an indicator of physiological stress. Cortisol does not increase when the infant is allowed to cry in its mother's arms, or in those of a substitute caregiver.

For all the fuss they make, babies don't actually begin shedding tears when they cry until they're about two months old. Before that they scream, which seems to work just as well. Researchers have discovered that prenatal crying also occurs. The fact that crying occurs in the womb suggests that it is not necessarily a learned behavior, although it obviously can be modified following birth by socialization, context, and relationships.[7]

Tears in History

Tears have faded in and out of fashion, and the differences with which they have been regarded are dramatic. For example, Homer has the Greek warrior Odysseus weeping in nearly every chapter of *The Iliad*; and when France's great medieval warrior Roland died, 20,000 knights wept so copiously they fainted and fell from their horses.[8] Emotional displays of this sort have become unthinkable on modern battlefields—can you imagine 20,000 sobbing, syncopal Marines?— or any place where high levels of discipline are valued.

Throughout the Middle Ages and well into the sixteenth century, it was considered appropriate for sensitive men and women alike to sob in public at a play, opera, or symphony. But with the advent of the Industrial Revolution, crying went out of favor. Factories needed focused, unemotional workers, not crybabies. Thus weeping became, for men, a private affair that took place behind closed doors, if at all.[9]

Disdain for tears continues. Political figures, in particular, sometimes pay a price for weeping in public. In 1972, Ed Muskie saw his presidential hopes dashed when he cried before cameras because of a critical report about his wife. If he couldn't handle his emotions, how could he be a good president? In 1987, Congresswoman Pat Schroeder was severely criticized for weeping in public when she withdrew from her run for the presidency.[10]

Saving Tears

Tears are so highly valued as an expression of love and caring they have often been collected and stored in bottlelike containers called lachrymatories. The practice is ancient. Ten centuries before the birth of Christ, in Psalms 56:8, David prays to God, "Thou tellest my wanderings: put thou my tears into thy bottle: are they not in thy book?" In the Roman era, mourners filled small tear bottles or cups with tears and placed them in tombs as a symbol of respect for the departed. The volume of tears attested to the status of the deceased individual; thus mourners were sometimes recruited and paid for the specific purpose of producing and collecting tears for these containers. Lachrymatories from the Roman period can be found today in museums around the world.

Tear bottles made a comeback during the Victorian era. During this time, bottles were made with special openings that permitted the tears of mourners to evaporate, and when they had done so the period of mourning was considered over. During the American Civil War, women collected their tears in small bottles as a sign of love for their men at war.

A lachrymatory renaissance is under way in the United States. For a modest price, skilled glassblowers will design and craft your personal tear bottle. You can even send in your tears to one glass artist, who will encase them in a glass teardrop that can be worn as a necklace, "so your tears can be close to your heart."[11]

Tearful Mysteries

One of the strangest cases I've ever come across is that of a 56-year-old Australian woman who shed tears from one eye at a time. If she thought of her mother, she wept freely only from her right eye, but if she thought of her father her tears would switch to the left eye. Her therapists dubbed her condition "alternating unilateral lachrymation." She was a victim of sexual abuse during childhood, and as an adult suffered periodic catatonic, trancelike states. The association of her father, the presumed source of abuse, with the left eye is interesting. Throughout history the left side is considered the "sinister" side, whence "sin" originates. After years of therapy, which consisted of counseling and hypnosis, she learned to cry from both eyes.[12,13]

As this case shows, mysteries abound where weeping is concerned. Experts can't even agree on why tears and crying originated in the first place.

Syndicated health columnist Judy Foreman is intrigued by tears. In her article "Sob Story," she assembles some exotic facts about them:[14]

• Before puberty, girls and boys cry the same amount, but by age 18 women cry considerably more.

- Men's and women's tear glands are structurally different, but nobody knows why.
- Normal tears are a three-layered film that lubricates the eye. The topmost mucin layer is made in the eyelid and on the surface of the eye. The watery or aqueous middle layer is secreted by the lachrymal gland above the eye. The topmost oily layer is made in the meibomian gland in the eyelid.
- Ten million Americans, mostly women, don't make enough tears and suffer from "dry eye." Androgen, a male hormone, and pro-lactin, a female hormone, promote healthy tears, and both hormones diminish with age. Androgen eye drops are being tested to see if they work better than over-the-counter artificial tears.
- Adults sob only once in every dozen crying episodes.
- Emotional tears are more protein-rich than irritant tears, such as the onion-slicing kind.
- Both emotional and irritant tears contain more than thirty times the amount of manganese found in the blood. This suggests that tears may function to rid the body of certain toxins. Indeed, in seabirds such as cormorants and albatrosses, tear glands seem to serve this purpose; they are more powerful than the birds' kidneys in ridding the body of toxic levels of salt.

Biochemist William Frey II, a leading tear researcher at the Ramsey Medical Center in Minneapolis, agrees that the ability to cry must have served a major function, or else it would not have persisted throughout the course of human evolution. Frey's favorite hypothesis is stress relief. "Science has proven that stress is terrible for the health of your brain, heart, and other organs," he says. "It isn't proven yet, but weeping has most likely served humans throughout our evolutionary history by reducing stress."

In a classic study,[15] Frey and his colleagues studied crying behaviors in five different groups of people for a month, asking them about emotional crying episodes and irritant weeping, such as from cutting onions. He asked them to record the date, time, duration, reason for crying, thoughts and emotions, and physical signs such as a lump in the throat, watery eyes, or flowing tears. He found that 94 percent of women had an emotional crying episode over the course of a month, compared to 55 percent of men. Of the women who cried, 85 percent said they felt better and more relieved after a good cry, as did 73 percent of the men. The duration of the crying episodes were the same in women and men, but Frey found that they cried differently. Women made lots of crying sounds, while men cried quietly as their eyes mainly brimmed with tears. Frey found that women cry on average 5.3 times a month, and men 1.4 times.

He also found that tears caused by irritants are 98 percent water, and that emotional tears contain more toxins than irritant tears. This suggests that one of the functions of crying may be to remove waste products from the body, and may help explain why people feel refreshed after crying.

"In just a few short decades, we've gone from the view that crying is just a loss of control and a sign of weakness to a common perception that there might be some value in open emotional crying," Frey says.[16] Dr. Barry M. Bernfeld, director of Los Angeles' Primal Institute, agrees. "Crying is natural, healthy and curative," he says. Still, there's a long way to go in its acceptance. "Crying," he observes, "which should be the most natural, accepted way of coping with pain, stress, and sorrow, is hardly mentioned in psychiatric literature." [17]

A Cry for Help

Infants cry as a way of communicating to their mothers that they are hungry, in pain, or are experiencing emotional distress, and they learn that crying gets results. This form of communication may carry over into adulthood, because crying, for adults, as for babies, is a highly effective way to draw another into one's orbit. When we see someone crying, we want to come to their aid. That's because crying "is a distress signal," says James Gross, Stanford University psychology professor. "This means that crying may be nature's way of forcefully signaling that we need help, and motivating helpful behavior designed to end tears and sadness."[18,19]

The cry-for-help hypothesis is affirmed by a team of Spanish ophthalmologists who analyzed 465 different crying episodes, searching for a common motivating factor behind the weeping.[20] "The only common factor in all tear-spilling episodes," they report, "was a relationship with help: either requesting help or offering help."

But why should seeking help have become paired with the act of shedding tears in our evolutionary past? It seems an odd connection when you think about it. Crying was selected, these researchers suggest, because it was handy; tearing was already present and established as a reflex response to physical pain when trauma and inflammation of the eyes occurred, as frequently happened in humankind's past. In other words, crying was already established as a signal that help was needed, so it was taken advantage of.

Crying as Healing

An important study of patients with rheumatoid arthritis (RA) suggests that we cry as a way of relieving chronic pain and inflammation.[21] Japanese researchers at Tokyo's Nippon Medical School exposed RA patients to deeply emotional stimuli, and correlated various neuroendocrine and immune responses (NEIRs) in their bodies with how easily they were brought to tears. These responses included blood levels of the stress hormone cortisol, the immune protein interleukin-6, and CD4, CD8, and natural killer immune cells. They found that patients who were easily moved to tears generally did better clinically over the course of a year than those who did not cry. The researchers concluded that shedding tears suppresses the influence of stress on their NEIRs, making their RA easier to control. This study goes against the grain of the grin-and-bear-it school, which says that pain and illness should be endured without complaint or whimper.

One of the most famous illnesses of the twentieth century was that of writer-publisher Norman Cousins, who used hysterical laughter as a therapy (among others) in turning around a life-threatening, painful, inflammatory illness thought to be ankylosing spondylitis.[22,23] Does Cousins' experience with laughter contradict the above findings about the value of easy crying? Perhaps not. Laughter and tears are obviously related, as when we say, "I laughed so hard I cried." It may turn out that it is deep emotion in general, not whether we specifically shed tears or laugh, that explains why inflammation and pain improve. Perhaps the body can't tell the difference between laughter and tears. If so, we can wonder whether Cousins might also have recovered if he had watched deeply sad movies that moved him to tears, instead of viewing laughter-producing comedies.

Evidence for the therapeutic benefit of weeping is a welcome finding. For years, enthusiasts of laughter and levity have promoted them as an intervention for nearly everything. A problem has been that laughter does not come easily for those suffering from acute and painful, chronic conditions. For them, weeping may be a more humane and effective recommendation.

People differ in their healing responses to every therapy. One size never fits all. "Laughter for some, tears for others" is likely to prove the best approach.

Tears and Health Care

Health-care professionals are usually considered unemotional, but surveys suggest otherwise. A 1997 Australian study examined the incidence of crying among doctors, nurses, and medical students, and found that 57 percent of doctors, 76 percent of nurses, and 31 percent of medical students had cried at work in the hospital at least once. The main reason given was the same for all three groups: "Identification and bonding with suffering and dying patients or their families."

Crying in health-care environments is not without cost. Medical students reported the highest percentage of negative consequences of their crying, such as being ridiculed or screamed at. And crying evokes guilt. A third of the respondents were troubled by their weeping responses, and said they were interested in or would consider psychological help in exploring their own emotional reactions to crying.

Because of the high frequency of crying among hospital staff, the researchers recommended that the subject of crying should be addressed in the training of physicians and nurses.[24]

Pathological Tears

The reasons people cry are extremely varied and sometimes indicate disease. One such condition is gelastic seizures, which are brief outbursts of emotion, usually in the form of laughing, shouting, or weeping. Jerking, stiff posturing, abnormal eye movements, and chewing or grinding of the teeth often accompany these symptoms. As with most seizures, the individual may be dazed or confused following the seizure.

People sometimes make too many tears—so-called crocodile tears or pathological lachrymation. Botox—the weakened form of botulinum toxin used to smooth out facial wrinkles—has come to the rescue of these individuals. In several studies, physicians have corrected the situation by injecting botulinum toxin directly into and around the lachrymal gland above the eye.[25,26,27]

(This isn't the only type of "weeping" botulinum toxin turns off. It's also used for too much armpit sweating, called "primary axillary hyperhidrosis." People who suffer from this condition produce up to five times the normal amount of armpit sweat, which can interfere greatly with normal social function. This situation is so disturbing that surgery is often employed to remove the sweat glands or to sever nerves in an attempt to paralyze the sweating mechanism. A single superficial injection of botulinum toxin, given once or twice a year, helps patients significantly.[28,29] Injections of botulinum toxin have also turned off another rare form of hypersecretion called Frey's syndrome or "gustatory sweating." This problem involves excessive warmth, flushing, or sweating in the cheekbone area of the face on eating, thinking, or talking about food.)

Any time crying or laughter occurs unprovoked or is generally devoid of emotional content, it should trigger suspicions of an underlying brain abnormality. A typical case involved a 46-year-old man who began to experience inappropriate crying, associated with spontaneous, uncontrollable laughter. He was aware that his labile emotions were not normal and had sought psychiatric help. He eventually developed weakness of the left side of his face and problems with balance. His neurological evaluation included an MRI brain scan, which showed a tumor at the back of his brain in the cerebellopontine angle. Surgery was successful, and his unprovoked crying spells and laughter stopped immediately following his operation.[30]

Pathological crying and laughter have also been reported in multiple sclerosis, traumatic brain injury, insecticide exposure, and stroke. Some cases have been immediately and permanently reversed by therapy with selective serotonin uptake inhibitors, of which Prozac is an example.[31]

Onion Tears

The most common tear-jerking experience in the world may be cutting onions. As Benjamin Franklin noted, "Onions can make even heirs and widows weep."[32] "Onion tears" are caused by sulfur-containing compounds in the vegetable that are liberated on cutting. These chemicals dissolve in the watery film over the eyes, creating a dilute solution of sulfuric acid that is irritating and tear-producing. Because these offending compounds are concentrated at the base of the onion, cutting off the root end last helps prevent onion tears.

Now Japanese food scientists are tinkering with an enzyme in onions they call lachrymatory-factor synthase, which produces the irritant responsible for onion tears.[33] Scientists everywhere are excited.

The Japanese discovery may "open up a new era of onion science and horticulture," enthuses organic chemist Eric Block, of State University of New York at Albany. But is it wise to change onions merely to eliminate cooks' tears? Maybe not. Block cautions, "It's reasonable to assume that Mother Nature incorporated the [tear-causing chemical] to afford some protection. An onion stripped of this defense may be more prone to attack by insects and microorganisms."[34] It's not nice to fool Mother Nature.

Onions have been credited as a source of health and strength through the ages. Greek athletes, prior to competing in the Olympic games, would consume pounds of onions, drink onion juice, and rub onions on their bodies. The Romans valued onions as a curative for a remarkable variety of illnesses, from dog bites to dysentery. When excavators unearthed Pompeii, they found cavities in the ground left by growing onions. By the Middle Ages, the three main vegetables of European cuisine had become beans, cabbage, and onions. The Pilgrims brought onions with them on the *Mayflower*, only to find them growing wild in abundance, and already being used by Native Americans as food and medicine.[35]

"Onion" is derived from the Latin *unio*, meaning oneness and unity.[36] Change the first "o" in onion to "u" and you've got "union," the achievement of which, with the Divine, has been the goal of spiritual seekers for millennia. It is not surprising, therefore, that reverence for onions abounds historically. Affirming this connection, the American author Charles Dudley Warner (1829–1900) said "The onion is the only vegetable that represents the essence of things. It can be said to have a soul."[37]

The ancient Egyptians agreed. They considered onions symbolic of eternity and buried them alongside their pharaohs. To them, eternal life was represented in the anatomy of the onion, with its concentric circles within a circle. Perhaps that is why King Ramses IV, who died in 1160 BCE, was embalmed with onions in his eye sockets.

Predictably, perhaps, cynical Westerners have seen it differently. As the American art critic James Gibbons Huneker (1860–1921) said,

"Life is like an onion; you peel off layer after layer and then you find there is nothing in it." Or as poet Carl Sandberg similarly complained, "Life is like an onion. You peel it off one layer at a time, and sometimes you weep."[38]

Scientists hoping to improve nature by fixing onions had better be careful lest they anger the onion gods, which seem to have been quite numerous. In Egyptian tomb paintings, onions appear on the altars of deities. Priests are depicted holding onion offerings in their hands.

In view of the onion's sobering history, perhaps we should hesitate to meddle with its inner workings. You never know when the mummy's curse might be unleashed.

So, a word of advice to you onion scientists. Back off, you guys. Show onions a little respect. We don't need to recalibrate their genome. All we need to do is put them in the fridge for a half hour or in the freezer for ten minutes before cutting them, leaving the root end till last.

And if this doesn't work, well, what's wrong with a few tears?

5

Dirt

Cleanliness is, indeed, next to godliness.

—JOHN WESLEY

Cleanliness is almost as bad as godliness.

— H. L. MENCKEN

I grew up on a small farm in central Texas. Like all the farm families in that part of the country, we depended on a deep well in the back yard for our drinking water. Drawing water was my chore, and one I always enjoyed—letting the bucket free-fall through the pulley, hearing it clank against the brick sides of the well before splashing 100 feet below in the cold, crystal-clear water, and drawing it up hand over hand.

One summer when I was about twelve years old, two events happened which initially seemed unrelated but which were intimately connected. First, the well water began to taste a bit strange; second, the family cat disappeared. We assumed he'd strayed until one day I drew up a bucket of water and noticed something furry. It was the cat—part of him, anyway. From the state of decomposition it was obvious he'd fallen into the well some time ago, which meant that for days we'd been drinking the water into which he was slowly dissolving.

My father, normally unflappable, decided that this was a potential medical crisis requiring immediate attention. He drove into town and returned with Dr. Riggs, the family doctor. Dr. Riggs was fiftyish, strikingly handsome, and arrived dressed in his customary white shirt, tie, and rolled-up sleeves. A visit from the doctor was a significant event, usually associated with a birth or death in the family, and this was no exception. As my father escorted Dr. Riggs to the well, I tagged along. Dad asked me to draw up a bucket of water for the doctor's inspection. I let the bucket linger at the bottom of the well to make sure I snagged a representative piece of the cat, which would impress the doctor with the seriousness of our predicament. When the water came up clear and furless, my heart sank. Dr. Riggs nonetheless bent over the bucket and gazed into it intently for a long time, like a shaman reading an oracle at a sacred well. Then, gathering himself, he declared with total confidence that everything looked fine—but, just to make sure, he'd take a water sample back to his office and "do a test." If we didn't hear from him in a week, we could resume drinking water from the well. His word was gospel in those parts, and our family trusted him implicitly. We hauled water from a neighboring farm for a week. Then, having heard nothing from the doctor, we began to drink the well water again, as if nothing had happened.

The situation took a terrible turn when, a few days later, I drew up a fresh bucket of water and saw the remains of a cat's paw floating on the surface. I realized that Dr. Riggs had been flat-out wrong in his assurances; the water obviously was still contaminated and my family was still at risk. I found myself in a dilemma. If I told the family about my discovery, Dr. Riggs would appear incompetent. But if I didn't confess, we would continue drinking the tainted water and might get sick. By the next day I had decided that Dr. Riggs's image needed more protection than my family's health. We'd weathered greater challenges than a drowned cat. So I decided to keep the information about the cat's paw to myself. It was the perfect decision. Nobody got sick, the cat eventually dissolved into oblivion, the water tasted better than ever, and Dr. Riggs seemed wise as always.

The drowned cat was only one among an endless chain of encounters with germs my brother, sister, and I experienced growing up.

Farm kids were exposed to microbial assaults on every hand—working in gardens and fields, drinking unpasteurized milk and contaminated water, swimming in stagnant water holes, and being perpetually scraped by tools and scratched by animals. Farm families in central Texas did not enjoy chlorinated water or indoor plumbing; these existed only in that distant domain we called "in town." Yet we farm kids were reaping an invisible dividend without realizing it. Our continual exposure to microbes was giving our immune system the workout it needed. Every day we faced microbial challenges similar to those encountered by humans during the millions of years they have lived close to the earth, animals, and each other. As a result, as we'll see, we farm kids got something our urban friends did not: a cast-iron resistance to disease.

Filth Phobia

Like farm families everywhere, my family was not skittish about a little dirt. As a result, I am often amused at the obsessions people often have about germs.

An example is tycoon Howard Hughes, whose eccentric health habits came to light following his death in 1976. Hughes had insisted on severing his contacts with people who had been his friends and acquaintances for months and years, fearing they would infect him if they became sick. By the summer of 1958 his phobia of germs drove him to seclusion in a hotel in Beverly Hills. Here the billionaire spent a great deal of his time sitting naked in a portion of his living room he designated the "germ-free zone," where he handled everything with tissue. "At one point," reports *New Scientist* writer Garry Hamilton, "he issued aides a three-page memo on the most hygienic way to open a tin of fruit."[1]

Hughes refused to touch doorknobs. He required his aides to wear gloves when passing objects to him and to write him messages rather than communicating verbally, which might spread germs. All doors and windows were sealed with tape to keep out dirt. He spent hours cleaning his phone with tissues. Here are the instructions he gave to his staff on how to remove a hearing aid cord from the cabinet in which it was stored:

> First use 6 or 8 thicknesses of Kleenex pulled one at a time from the slot in touching the door knob to open the door to the bathroom. The door is to be left open so there will be no need to touch anything when leaving the bathroom. The same sheaf of Kleenex may be employed to turn on the spigots so as to obtain a good force of warm water. This Kleenex is then to be disposed of. The hands are to be washed with extreme care, far more thoroughly than they have ever been washed before, taking great pains that the hands do not touch the sides of the bowl, the spigots, or anything else in the process.[2]

Hughes was involved in a death struggle against germs and dirt, and in the end the dirt won. When he became constipated he would spend up to twenty-six hours in the bathroom, sometimes urinating on the floor or against the bathroom door. He forbade his staff to clean up the mess, preferring instead to spread towels on the floor. He began to take all sorts of medications as protection against disease. In spite of his terrors, he was amazingly capable of conducting business. But toward the end he began to spend more time in bed, rarely bathed, and let his finger- and toenails grow long. Emaciated and deranged from following a frugal diet and taking too many drugs, Hughes died while flying from Acapulco to Houston for medical treatment.[3]

"Such behavior is irrational by anybody's standards, but don't we all have a little Howard Hughes inside us?" asks Hamilton. "After all, we can now wipe our antibacterial cutting board with an antibacterial sponge, shower with antibacterial soap, and sleep beneath an antibacterial quilt on an antibacterial pillow. In Japan, you can even bank with an antibacterial deposit book, and soon, according to reports, drive to work in a car fitted with an antibacterial steering wheel."[4]

A Dirty Little Healing

When my book *Healing Words: The Power of Prayer and the Practice of Medicine* was published in 1993, it stirred a great deal of interest in the popular media.[5] One of the major television networks dispatched a crew to Santa Fe to film an interview with me about prayer's role in conventional medicine. For the site of the interview we chose an old adobe Catholic church twenty-four miles northeast of Santa Fe— El Santuario de Chimayó.

Sometime around 1810 in Chimayó, a humble friar discovered a crucifix buried on a hillside, to which he had been led by a luminous light bursting forth from the earth. A local priest tried to relocate the crucifix three times, but each time it was discovered back in its original hole, as if it wanted to remain there. A small chapel was built on the site in honor of this seemingly miraculous event. Around 1816 the chapel was expanded into the current adobe sanctuary, which is considered a classic in Spanish colonial church architecture.

Miraculous healings began to be reported from the location almost as soon as the crucifix was discovered. They became connected with El Posito, the "sacred sand pit" in which the cross was believed to have originated. The curative powers of the sacred dirt have become legendary. Each year thousands of pilgrims come from all over the world to take away a little of the dirt, much like people travel to Lourdes in France to obtain water from the sacred spring in the hope of being healed. In fact, El Santuario de Chimayó is called the Lourdes of the Southwest. And as at Lourdes, the walls of the sacristy are hung with discarded crutches and other objects as evidence that something remarkable happens here.

The camera crew and I arrived at the shrine late in the afternoon. There was a serious problem: The host of the show was recovering from a cold and sore throat. A minute into his monologue that introduced the interview, he would begin coughing and would have to start all over. He tried half a dozen times to deliver his introduction, with no success. The film crew was anxious; the sun was setting and soon they would be unable to finish the assignment. The project was headed for disaster.

Then I thought, why not take advantage of the healing power of the sacred dirt of Chimayó? Having nothing to lose, I asked the camera crew to take a break while I dashed into the sacristy and scooped up a handful of the stuff. Then I returned to the interviewer and asked his permission to apply it to his throat, just as pilgrims for two centuries have applied it to the part of the body that needed healing. Although I am sure he doubted my sanity, the host was a good sport and let me rub the dirt onto his neck from chin to sternum. Then I dusted it off, rearranged his shirt, and asked him to do his monologue once again. By this time the camera crew were rolling their eyes, irritated that I had wasted more time. But on the very next take the host completed his monologue without coughing—and just to make sure his improvement was for real, he did two additional takes, both flawless. His voice was getting stronger, and we had a fine interview. Unfortunately, the cameras weren't rolling when I had applied the dirt to his neck, so this dirt-mediated healing was not captured on film. It would have been a perfect example of the program's focus.

Germ Consciousness

Where did our fear of germs come from?

A little more than a century ago, ordinary folk in America had no idea that the diseases that often killed them and their children were related to microorganisms. The phrase "germ theory of disease" did not come into common use in the English-language medical literature until around 1870, writes Nancy Tomes, professor of history at the State University of New York at Stony Brook in her admirable book *The Gospel of Germs: Men, Women, and the Microbe in American Life.*[6] The idea that germs are actually evil became fixed in the modern mind on the heels of Darwinism in the second half of the nineteenth century. Although Darwin spoke of life-and-death struggles in nature and of survival of the fittest, he did not moralize about these processes.

Many of his contemporaries, however, were not as cautious. Tomes describes how many naturalists saw a conscious malevolence in disease-causing germs. These scientists used lurid terms to describe microbes, such as "foreign," "base," "murderous," and "cunning." It was as if the germs were doing bad things on purpose, and the idea of invisible killers terrified people. Gradually, "germ consciousness" took root.[7]

Examples that germs could kill were everywhere and no one was safe. Typhoid killed President Abraham Lincoln's beloved son, as well as Queen Victoria's husband. Theodore Roosevelt's mother succumbed to the disease on the same day his wife died in childbirth.

The death of Roosevelt's mother at age 48 in New York City from one of the "filth diseases," as they were coming to be called, is a poignant example of the fear and helplessness people felt.[8] Although no one knew the specific causal agents, these were illnesses known to be spread by fecal contamination. As such, they were considered preventable by proper domestic sanitation. By all accounts, Martha Bulloch Roosevelt, known familiarly as "Mittie," was so concerned about cleanliness that her friends thought her almost obsessive. The mansion the Roosevelts occupied on West Fifty-Seventh Street had been built by Theodore Senior in the 1870s, and had been designed by the leading architects of the day and incorporated the latest advances in sanitation-related fixtures. Mittie had moved from rural Georgia to New York City after her marriage in 1853 and was appalled at the filth of the rapidly growing city. Special measures were required to combat it. These included a daily bath with two changes of water, spreading a sheet on the floor at night when she said her prayers, and wearing white clothing even in winter, to make sure that no speck of dirt escaped detection. Assisted by her small army of servants, she kept her house as clean as herself. She compiled a lengthy set of housekeeping instructions including a rigorous program of polishing, scrubbing, sweeping, and dusting. When the ash man came each morning, for example, the cook was required to greet him with a bucket of scalding water to decontaminate his ash can before he could enter the house.

"Such a fastidious woman would surely have died of shame," says Tomes, "had the typhoid fever not killed her, to discover that she had contracted a disease spread by fecal contamination. Martha Roosevelt's death from typhoid epitomized the uncertainties that beset even the most conscientiously clean households of the Gilded Age: no one, not even the most careful, seemed to be safe from the invisible agents of disease."[9]

In the nineteenth century, rates of illness and death rose sharply in the large cities of America and Europe, making them dangerous places to live. To survive, as Martha Roosevelt's death showed, you had to be not only clean, but tough and lucky as well. It wasn't just the periodic epidemics of cholera and smallpox that people endured, there were also endemic diseases such as typhoid and pneumonia which killed at a steady rate, year after year. In the 1880s in New York City, one-fifth of all infants died before reaching their first birthday, often of infant diarrhea, and even if they reached adulthood, they had a one-in-four chance of succumbing between the ages of twenty and thirty.[10] Death and germs stalked everyone, all the time. Before long, the dangers of the "Three D's"—dirt, disease, and death—were being hammered into the American psyche."[11]

Cellophane and Listerine

By the time the nineteenth century wound down, germ consciousness had become deeply rooted in the American psyche. Money was to be made.

In 1908, a Swiss chemist invented a flexible cellulose film, which was acquired in 1923 by the Du Pont Company and named Cellophane. Du Pont improved the product by making it more moisture-proof and less expensive, and marketed it to industries such as those producing candy, baked goods, and processed meats. To the public, Du Pont emphasized Cellophane's role in germ protection. Cellophane ads warning ominously of the dangers of the deadly trio of "flies, fingers, and food" soon appeared in the *Saturday Evening Post*,

Good Housekeeping, and *Ladies' Home Journal.* The *Cellophane Radio Show* aired in the morning right before housewives went shopping, and featured etiquette expert Emily Post.[12]

In the 1920s, ads for Listerine—named after Joseph Lister, who introduced antisepsis into surgery—began to feature pretty young women whose hopes for a happy marriage were ruined because of "halitosis," which the ad men represented as a horrid condition caused by mouth bacteria. Using Listerine could help one avoid the stigma of "always a bridesmaid, never a bride." Listerine was also marketed for use as an undiluted handwash. One ad informed the reader about "17 diseases carried by the hands . . . many of them dangerous." Another ad was directed at mothers: "If you could look at your hands under a microscope you would hesitate to prepare or serve baby's food, or give him a bath, without first rinsing the hands with undiluted Listerine." Using these approaches, Lambert Pharmacal Company's sales went from $100,000 in 1920 to $4 million just seven years later.[13]

Disposability

Germ consciousness also paved the way for the idea of disposability. Eighty thousand tons of toilet tissue were produced in 1919, the first year it was listed as a separate area of manufacture. In 1935, paper cup manufacturers established the Cup and Container Institute, which warned of the dangers of unsterile drinking glasses and the "mutualization of saliva" while traveling and eating out, which could be avoided by demanding paper drinking cups and plates.[14]

Germs and the Lord's Supper

A little-known skirmish in the nineteenth-century wars between science and religion took place as a direct result of the growing uneasiness over germs, and concerned the common communion cup used in Protestant churches.[15] Physicians charged that the cup had been implicated in the transmission of not only tuberculosis but also "loathsome diseases" too foul to name, and suggested that the practice be abandoned. Their proposal met with stiff resistance among the faithful. Many Protestants countered that if the common cup was good enough for Jesus and his disciples, it was good enough—and safe enough—for them. The arguments raged. When the Walnut Street Presbyterian Church in Philadelphia voted in 1898 to shift to an individual-cup system, churches throughout the country followed suit, including Baptists, Congregationalists, Lutherans, Methodists, Presbyterians, and Universalists.[16]

The Hygiene Hypothesis

Today, an ironic development is taking place in the battle against germs. A growing number of researchers are suggesting that our increasing separation from dirt and microbes carries a serious price tag and may, in fact, be killing us. Their proposal is called the "hygiene hypothesis"—the basic idea being that too much cleanliness is bad for you, that we *need* germs.

Throughout most of humankind's evolutionary history, we were continually assailed with dirt and microbes from the moment of birth. Our immune system evolved sophisticated chemical pathways and a variety of specialized immune cells to protect us. If these challenges to the immune system are removed, as they largely have been in modern times, things backfire. To illustrate, scientists suggest an analogy from infancy. If a baby is raised without affection and social contact, its brain cells fail to make the right connections and the infant grows up mentally or emotionally impaired. Similarly, adults go into mental decline when they fail to receive proper intellectual and emotional stimulation. In the same way, our immune system fails to develop properly if it is not given the challenges it requires in our earliest days.[17]

Immunologist Graham Rook of University College, London, is an enthusiastic proponent of the hygiene hypothesis. Rook suggests that vaccines, which are designed to confer immunity artificially, are a poor substitute for immunity that is acquired naturally. Vaccines over-stimulate one branch of the immune system, he maintains, and this imbalance may underlie the epidemic rise in asthma in the United States, Western Europe, Japan, and Australia. For example, in Britain and Australia, between 20 and 30 percent of the population suffers from asthma, while this condition was unusual only 30 years ago. In the United States, five thousand people die every year from this dis-ease, in spite of increasingly effective medications. Hay fever and eczema are also rampant.

Modernization and wealth were supposed to lead to increases in health, and in many ways they have, evidenced by the increase in longevity during the previous century in industrialized countries. But conundrums abound. We have recently attributed the cause of asthma, for example, to dirty air. But in the United States, although the air is becoming cleaner, the incidence of asthma is increasing and asthma and allergies are more common in Sweden's southern cities, where the air is relatively clean, when compared with certain cities in Poland. Some experts tried to explain the rising incidence of asthma and allergies to an increase in house dust mites, but the numbers of mites actually leveled off years ago.[18]

Family Size

In 1989, David Strachan, an epidemiologist at the London School of Hygiene and Tropical Diseases, noticed that kids growing up with lots of siblings had a lower incidence of asthma, hay fever, and child-hood eczema.[19] He hypothesized that older siblings might be bring-ing home all sorts of infections and spreading them around, which somehow benefited their brothers and sisters. "Over the past century declining family size, improvements in household amenities, and higher standards of personal cleanliness have reduced the opportu-nity for cross infection in young families," Strachan stated in the *British Medical Journal.* "This may have resulted in more widespread clinical expression of [allergylike] disease, emerging earlier in wealthier people. . . ."[20] The idea was heresy when Strachan advanced it in 1989, because infections were then believed to *trigger* allergy-related illnesses, not protect from them.

But yesterday's heresies have a way of becoming today's science, and other researchers are beginning to agree with Strachan's basic idea. In one study in the West African nation of Guinea-Bissau, teenagers and young adults who contracted measles during a 1979 epidemic are now only half as likely to have allergies as those who escaped the disease.[21,22] And another study found that Italian military students with antibodies to hepatitis A, having contracted the disease in the past, have allergies that are less common and less severe than students lacking these antibodies.[23]

Skeptics suggest that children who fight off measles and who develop hepatitis A antibodies have immune systems that are more fit to begin with. And in many inner cities in the United States, where kids live in crowded conditions and experience repeated infections early in life, they still have an extremely high asthma rate.[24] Therefore the challenge for researchers is to find a smoking gun—evidence that having an infection at a particular point in life actually switches off an allergic sensitization reaction.

Reverse Quarantine

When I was young, parents often deliberately exposed their young children to kids in other households who were sick with mumps, measles, and chicken pox. My siblings and I considered this cruel and unusual punishment—being hauled to a distant farmhouse and being forced to play or chat with friends with strange rashes, sores, or swellings. When we were sick with one of these infections, we could be certain our friends would visit us. The purpose behind this reverse quarantine was to spread these childhood viral infections, because of the belief that if one acquired them while young they were more benign than in adulthood.

Long before the hygiene hypothesis was elaborated, these farm families embodied a version of it in their folk wisdom. They understood that childhood sickness could promote long-term health, and that one sometimes needs to cooperate with illness instead of fighting it. What a contrast with current child-rearing practices, in which parents often do everything possible to *prevent* their children from getting sick.

Evidence suggests that the folk wisdom was correct. Researcher Anne-Louise Ponsonby of the Australian National University and her colleagues examined whether children exposed to siblings two years old or younger during the first six years of life had a reduced risk of multiple sclerosis (MS) as they grew older.[25] A viral cause for MS has long been considered, and researchers have long suspected that early life infections may make an individual less susceptible to it.[26] Ponsonby's team found that high exposure to very young siblings was indeed correlated with a lower risk of MS, as well as infectious mononucleosis, later in life.

The implications for day care are profound. Over 50 percent of preschool kids in the United States are in day care. Many parents are horrified at the idea of exposing their preschooler to the stew of germs that is always present in day-care settings. But if the payoff is a stronger immune system later in life, as the above research suggests, day care may be an excellent long-term health strategy for kids. Commitment to day care can be a difficult choice for working parents; perhaps the potential health benefits that are involved can make it less so.

Getting Dirty

Rook and his colleague John L. Stanford suggest that people's exposure, when growing up, to specific bacteria that are actually contained in the dirt is important. Mycobacteria have been the focus of a lot of their attention. These microbes abound in soil and in pond and stream water but not in the human body. When we began chlorinat-

ing water on a massive scale, we radically changed our exposure to
mycobacteria. In developing countries that do not chlorinate their
water supplies, there may be as many as one billion mycobacteria per
liter, whereas in the chlorine-treated waters of the West, the numbers
are negligible.[27]

When Rook and Wang injected mice with a vaccine made of
Mycobacterium vaccae, they suppressed the production of a substance
called serum immunoglobulin E (IgE), which is known to mediate
allergic response in humans.[28] Moreover, the injection stopped the
allergic response once it had started. Currently, British studies are in
progress to assess whether this procedure could be used therapeutically in humans with asthma and hay fever.

So Rook suggests that we may not be exposed to enough dirt, or
to the microbes dirt and dirty water contain. The problem, he says, is
that "the inner city guys don't have gardens." [29] Stanford adds, "The
change began right back in the Middle Ages. People moved away
from living in houses with dirt floors and started having reasonable
clothing and bathing and all the things that separate us from the environment. The excessive hygiene methods we now follow are yet
another step separating us from the essential learning process that the
immune system needs."[30]

Rook and his colleagues are not romanticizing filth, and they are
not suggesting that we abandon immunizations and start drinking
dirty, unchlorinated water. They are suggesting, however, that advances
in cleanliness come with a price and that we need to consider ways
around the problems caused by excessive hygiene. "If in the course of
everyday life, we don't meet enough bacteria," Rook says, "we're just
going to have to inject them ourselves."[31]

"If proponents of the hygiene hypothesis are correct," Hamilton
states, "of course, it will mean more than a new set of vaccines. Western society will also have to rethink its obsessive hatred of germs.
And while this obviously won't mean putting out the welcome mat
for bubonic plague, it might mean accepting that a little bit of dirt is
more of a tonic than you think."[32]

Dirt Remembered

In spite of our professed aversion to dirt, we humans can't shake its pull. Sometimes it seems that we want to merge with dirt.

Left alone, children eat dirt, as if hearkening to some atavistic urge, and they make mud pies before they are taught by hygienic parents that nice children don't get dirty. Like children, adults eat dirt occasionally, a practice called geophagia, and willingly pay considerable sums of money to be slathered from eyeballs to toenails with semiliquid dirt, a ritual called a mud bath. And there is the peculiar spectacle of mud wrestling, in which men and women shed every ounce of decorum and slither aggressively into the muck like angry earthworms. One of the most emblematic scenes of the uninhibited 1960s occurred at Woodstock, New York, in 1969, when thousands of ecstatic hippies frolicked in the mud, after rains turned Yasgur's farm into ankle-deep muck. In keeping with today's more subdued tone, millions experience the pleasures of dirt vicariously through characters such as Pigpen in Charles Schulz's "Peanuts" comic strip. Youngsters are similarly charmed by Oscar the Grouch of *Sesame Street*, who resides in a trash can.

What is going on here? Perhaps a clue to dirt's eternal appeal can be found in the etymology of "mud"—an Indo-European root from which "mother" is also derived: thus the maternal, intrauterine connotation of the dictionary's definition of mud as "wet, soft, sticky earth."[33] These nurturing, protective, maternal qualities may help explain why people the world over encase themselves in mud when constructing shelters, as if they are expressing a primordial urge to return to the womb.

I live in Santa Fe, New Mexico, a small town that was originally built totally of mud—earthen bricks mixed with brush or straw, called adobe.[34] When the Pueblo Native Americans originally employed these methods here, they made sense, because few building materials were to be found in this arid region. But even today, when cheaper and better construction materials are available, people still prefer adobe. The reason, they say, is that adobe is more attractive and authentic, truer to the history of the region. But I suspect the real reason they prefer living like cliff swallows, encased by mud, runs deeper.

Manners

The evolution of mannerly behavior can be seen as an attempt to clean up yet another side of life. A major step in sanitizing the dirty, messy side of eating occurred with the development of table manners. In 1972, Antoine de Courtin wrote a book of manners in which he declared it impolite to touch with the fingers anything greasy, a sauce, or syrup. This act was considered so repellent that those witnessing it could be expected to experience nausea. A napkin is crucial, otherwise one might be tempted to wipe the fingers on one's bread, or, what is worse, to lick them.[35]

"Impolite" is from the Latin *impolitus*, unpolished. To polish something is to scrub it clean of dirt and filth. The effect of polite table manners, therefore, was to polish the act of eating by eliminating the touching of food. The fork became allied with the napkin as a barrier to food. One wonders whether disposable gloves, which are increasingly being used by cooks and food servers today, will find their way to the table as further insulation against food. The barrier to food has become nearly absolute; not only do we not have to touch our food, we don't even have to look at it. We can buy liquid food and drink in a can, and drink them without every laying eyes on the stuff.

Vulgarity and Obscenity

Jungian analyst and author Clarissa Pinkola Estés suggests that a little dirt in the form of obscenity and vulgarity is good for the psyche. "The obscene is not vulgar at all," she contends in her best-selling book *Women Who Run with the Wolves*.[36] She notes that the word "obscene" comes from the old Hebrew *Ob*, meaning a wizard or sorceress. "There is an aspect of women's sexuality that in ancient times was called the sacred obscene, not in the way we use the word today, but meaning sexually wise in a witty sort of way. There were once goddess cults devoted to irreverent female sexuality. They were not derogatory, but concerned with portraying parts of the unconscious that remain, even today, mysterious and largely uncharted."[37]

Estés began telling "dirty goddess stories" in her workshops. "It became clear to me," she says, "that the importance of these old goddesses of obscenity was in their ability to loosen what was too tight, to lift gloom, to bring the body into a kind of humor that belongs not to the intellect but to the body itself, to keep these passages clear. . . . The obscene goddesses cause a vital form of neurological and endocrine medicine to spread throughout the body."[38]

The Shadow

Depth psychologists suggest that our repudiation of physical dirt parallels, on a psychological level, our rejection of those personal traits we consider to be unflattering, dark, evil, "dirty." These qualities are repressed into the unconscious, where they constitute "the shadow." But even though we may chase these qualities off the stage of awareness, they can't be wiped away as handily as physical dirt. They lurk in the hidden corners of the mind of everyone, where they exert powerful effects.

One way in which we distance ourselves from our distasteful personal qualities is by projecting these same traits onto others. When we project our hatred, for example, onto others, we often employ the vocabulary of germ consciousness—*dirty* Jews, the *plague* of conservatism or liberalism, the *infection* of moral depravity, whatever flavor our bigotry runs to.

Throughout history, rituals evolved as a way of acting out and neutralizing the dirt of the shadow, thus functioning as a kind of safety valve for the psyche. These rituals were bawdy, relatively innocuous, and fun. For centuries the Church didn't make much headway in its attempts to clean up the behavior of parishioners.

They were still trying to sanitize things when, in 1444, the Theological Faculty of Paris issued a letter to all the French bishops fulminating against festivals known as "Fools' Holidays." Even the priests joined in these celebrations, in which worshippers gleefully elect a "Fools' Pope," which was a deliberate insult to His Holiness. These events must have been quite a show. "[In] the very midst of divine service masqueraders with grotesque faces, disguised as women, lions and mummers, performed their dances, sang indecent songs in the choir, ate their greasy food from a corner of the altar near the priest celebrating mass, got out their games of dice, burned a stinking incense made of old shoe leather, and ran and hopped about all over the church."[39]

It's difficult to imagine such things happening in church these days. But the old urges remain, evidenced by the epidemic of unseemly behavior among the clergy—illicit sexual affairs, child molestation, and so on. We can wonder if the clergy would be better off acknowledging their pollution and devising ways of expressing it. Should Fools' Holidays be reinstated? Jung warned that unless we want to be broadsided by forbidden urges welling up from the unconscious, we must acknowledge all we are, warts and all. As philosopher Ken Wilber put it, we will *be aware* of our shadow, or we will *beware* it. The idea that "dirt belongs" is dramatically exemplified in Christianity, in Jesus' birth in a humble stable among unclean animals, and in his fraternization with dirty people from the margins of society such as crude fishermen and prostitutes.

The Trickster

The value of pollution is also echoed in trickster myths, which are found worldwide. The trickster is especially highly developed in Native American lore, where he appears as a coyote, raven, hare, and spider. He is a half-animal, half-divine prankster who revels in gluttony and sex. A traitor to germ theory, he often luxuriates in dirt and filth. Jung, who studied trickster myths extensively, believed that the irreverent customs that sprang up in the European churches of the Middle Ages, noted above, paralleled the trickster myths to perfection.[40]

There are also parallels in many healing traditions between the trickster and the healer. According to these beliefs, it is improper for healers to be too pure and perfect, for this separates them from those they serve. As Harvard's Eugene Taylor points out, "The *curandero* at the end of the trance ceremony smokes a cigarette. The purpose is to come back, to pollute himself so he can return to the world of others."[41] The warning of excessive perfection also appears in Greek mythology in the image of the "wounded healer" whose imperfections paradoxically make him or her more powerful.

Illness: Sitting with Our Dirt

Writer Kat Duff has given a powerful account of her long bout with chronic fatigue and immune deficiency syndrome (CFIDS) in her book *The Alchemy of Illness.* For years she experienced recurring fevers, incapacitation, aching muscles, extreme weakness, and memory loss. At one point in her illness she sank so deeply into despair she could not climb out of it. She hated life and behaved spitefully to her friends. She felt "small, dirty, and tainted," she says. Finally she "decided to stop complaining and just sit with my dirt." This proved a breakthrough. Her dreams began to give her guidance, including the vision that her faith must be practiced, and she began to pray daily. One dream told her to make a place for her "pack of black dogs . . . despair, envy, and hate . . . at the end of her bed."[42] An antidepressant helped as well.

In sitting with her dirt, Duff was honoring a principle of alchemical philosophy—that all things are related to their opposites, and that healing comes from the integration of the disparate elements of experience. In the aftermath of illness, she pondered why this principle is not more widely known. She believes that people don't discuss this side of their illness following recovery, because in time they resume their place among the healthy and either forget or repress the value of engaging the dark side of being sick. On getting well, we want to put these experiences behind us and move on. And who among the healthy would want to listen to these reports anyway? Thus the lesson of sitting with one's dirt during illness is not transmitted, and must always be rediscovered.[43]

Yet, "Only those people who really can touch bottom can be human," Jung emphasized.[44] But to touch bottom is to become even dirtier, because the bottom is where the muck lies. But as Duff found out, therein lies deliverance. Only when she hit bottom was her dirt transformed, and she began to heal.

This sort of talk, I've discovered, doesn't go over very well these days. Everywhere the premium is on "taking control," "exercising self-responsibility," and "creating your own reality," not sitting in your dirt and confronting the dark side of disease. The desire to look on the bright side permeates our culture in general. "Americans don't like tragedy," writer Martha Bayles states. "No matter how complex and heavy a problem, we get our social scientists to give it a name, divide it into stages, and suggest a method for working it through. Then we get our media to publicize the method, and pretty soon there's a 1-800 number to call as an alternative to despair."[45]

There is a tendency in everyone not only to reject our own dirt, but to denounce it in other people as well. This can lead to disastrous problems in human relationships. If we have no tolerance for what we consider to be the polluted ideas and behaviors of others, we are likely to force our personal standards of "cleanliness" on them—our ethics, morals, religion, even our personal beliefs about health care.

If we want to coexist peacefully, we shall have to acknowledge the dirt that exists both in ourselves and in others. And in rubbing shoulders with those whose dirt we don't approve of, we needn't worry too much about being contaminated by them. As Diogenes the Cynic said in the fourth century BCE, "The sun too penetrates into privies, but is not polluted by them."[46]

One day when I was on duty in a hospital emergency room, an ambulance arrived with a patient who had committed suicide. He was a diabetic man who had injected himself intravenously with an over-dose of insulin in the large vein at the bend of the elbow. By his arm the paramedics found a bottle of alcohol and a cotton sponge, with which he had sterilized the injection site before killing himself. Even though he knew he would die, he did not want to risk getting an infection. This memory has stayed with me over the years as an example of how our fears of uncleanness haunt us to the grave.

Our clinics, hospitals, and doctors' offices reinforce our concerns. Our images of them are of sparkling countertops and glassware, ster-ile, crystal-clear IV solutions, and immaculate, stainless-steel surgical instruments. And all hospitals are permeated with that ubiquitous antiseptic smell, an invisible talisman against infections. But sterility is only part of the equation of healing. As we have seen, evidence continues to mount for the value of the unclean and the unsanitary, particularly in our early years when our immune system is struggling toward maturity. As a result of these findings, health begins to seem like a magnet, which requires both a positive and negative pole to function.

In cities around the world, we find statues honoring the contribu-tions of individuals who waged war successfully against infections and uncleanness—Pasteur, Nightingale, Lister, Koch, Fleming, Salk, and scores of others. Yet there is not even a simple plaque anywhere that honors the contributions that a bacterium, fungus, virus, or just plain dirt make to our immune system—contributions without which *none* of us would be alive.

During the early years of my maternal grandparents' marriage, my grandfather, a farmer, journeyed from their home in central Texas to the southern part of the state in search of agricultural opportunities. In the course of his travels he visited Mexico. When he returned home he brought my grandmother a gift—a small, clear, glass bottle filled with something utterly precious, the value of which they both understood: *dirt*, which he had collected from a Mexican farm.

As a small child I was unable to understand why my grandfather chose such a gift. He died before I was born, so I never had the chance to ask him his reasons. But I was fascinated by the bottle and would turn it upside down endlessly, watching the sandy earth run from one end to the other, like an hourglass. There was magic here. Dirt had me in thrall.

Dirt meant more to my grandparents and my parents than a medium in which to grow crops, although they probably would have considered such a view grandiose and would have been embarrassed to hear me say so. Although they were no-nonsense farmers, their blood whispered to them dirt's value in all its nuances—physical, psychological, spiritual. Such knowledge used to be commonplace. In our urban paranoia of dirt and dirtiness, however, we have lost that awareness, and all the antibiotics and antiseptics in the world will not substitute for it.

Can we set aside our squeamishness and declare a truce on dirt? Can we make a place for the lowly, the humble, the unclean? If so, we might find that it is not just our immune system that benefits. A richer vision of "the unclean" just might translate into a deeper caring for the down-and-out unfortunates who struggle on the margins of society in every country in the world, including our own.

This change in emphasis does not require new knowledge, but a remembering. At some deep level we know the value of pollution—the grain of sand that stimulates the oyster to produce a beautiful pearl, the dust that makes a more beautiful sunset, and maybe, even, that damned cat in the well.

6

Music

A bird does not sing because it has an answer.
It sings because it has a song.

—*CHINESE PROVERB*

Sex commands more Internet listings than any other item—185 million, according to my recent Googling—and music isn't far behind. This reflects the fact that sex and music are two of the most potent influences on human behavior known—so powerful that institutions and governments have long tried to regulate them.

In *The Republic,* Plato stressed two factors, gymnastics and music, as essential in educating boys into the type of adults who would form the basis of an ideal society. But he realized that music can be tricky. "When a man abandons himself to music, he begins to melt and liquefy," he said. Therefore, not just any sort of music would do, but only that played in the respectable Dorian and Phrygian modes. If boys listened to the Lydian or Ionian forms,[1] they could be corrupted, because this music was "soft, lazy, and fit for drunkenness." Plato also considered these musical forms "useless even for women if they are to be decent." Socrates agreed. He advocated banning most of the musical modes or scales, "because more than anything else rhythm and harmony find their way to the inmost soul and take strongest hold upon it, bringing with them and imparting grace, if one is rightly trained, and otherwise the contrary."[2]

The Greeks also worried about the effects of music on the state. As Damon of Athens expressed this concern, "Musical modes are nowhere altered without changes in the most important laws of the state."[3] The anxieties of the Greeks about the fallout of music have cast long shadows. Political leaders continue to fret about the power of music to lead citizens astray and interfere with the smooth workings of the government.

Consider the Taliban regime, a collection of former theology students who ascended to power following the 1989 exit of the Soviets from Afghanistan. The "Tali-banners" hated fun and excelled at its prohibition. Almost all forms of recreation that brought joy to Afghan women, men, and children—movies, photography, dancing, even kite flying—were declared unlawful. Women's shoes that made noisy clicks were banned; such sounds could prove seductive. Goons from the Ministry of Promotion of Virtue and Prevention of Vice patrolled the streets of Kabul looking for infractions, and violators were beaten and sometimes executed.

Listening to music was considered particularly sinister. The Taliban engaged in search-and-destroy missions for musical instruments and cassette players and burned them on public pyres. As a warning, wooden poles at checkpoints were entwined with tangles of confiscated audiotape and film, flapping in the breeze. Musicians caught playing were beaten with their own instruments and imprisoned for up to forty days. The Taliban claimed that the Prophet had warned people to avoid listening to music lest molten lead be poured into their ears on the Day of Judgment. Religious songs and patriotic chants were exempted, provided they were not accompanied by musical instruments, and were played repeatedly on the state-run Radio Shariat. The archives of traditional Afghan folk songs at Kabul Radio were ransacked and destroyed.

The Taliban were hardly original. As journalist Richard Taruskin says, "All the enemies of music, like the Taliban, fear it has power over the soul. They're absolutely right."[4] Thus the Ayatollah Ruhollah Khomeini banned music from Iranian radio and television in 1979, likening its effects to opium—"stupefying persons listening to it and making their brains inactive and frivolous."[5]

Crackdowns on music are common wherever repressive regimes are found. Journalist Nadya Labi reports, "In the Sudan, musicians cannot perform after dark; in a Nigerian state where Islamic law is followed, a musician was recently imprisoned for singing. . . . [In Pakistan], shopkeepers sell cassettes on the black market, musicians bury their instruments for retrieval later, and drivers blare their stereos in remote areas."

Why are governments in the developing world phobic about music? "In much of the Third World, people cannot read or write," observes Marie Korpe, executive director of Freemuse, a Danish group that monitors censorship of music. "People listen to the radio, to songs. It is music that reaches people's hearts and souls."[6]

Western religions have also been skittish about music for a very long time.[7] It could distract people from more important things, such as theological issues. As Alexander Pope put it in 1711 in *An Essay on Criticism*, ". . . some to church repair,/Not for the doctrine, but the music there."[8] St. Augustine lamented in the fourth century that, as a result of the melodies he heard in church, "I have become a problem unto myself." Terrified of the connection between music and sex, John of Salisbury fretted in the twelfth century that the lofty music sung in the Cathedral of Notre Dame in Paris might "more easily occasion titillation between the legs than a sense of devotion in the brain." Books containing "popish ditties" were zealously burned in England and Switzerland by Protestant reformers. Later, musical instruments were burned by the Orthodox patriarch of Moscow because they were believed to lead to paganism. Sometimes fear of music is linked to fear of the female, writes Taruskin.[9] St. John Chrysostom, Father of the Greek Orthodox Church, warned that when marriages were celebrated, "dancing, and cymbals and flutes, and shameful words and songs from the lips of painted girls" were a conduit for "all the Devil's great heap of garbage."

In the United States, the public debate about censorship of music and the arts oscillates between extremes. Some advocate an "anything goes" policy in which musicians and artists are given a completely free rein. Others favor federal and state censorship designed to protect the morals and sensibilities of the citizenry, based almost always in a religious interpretation of right and wrong, good and evil.

If you doubt the power of music to mold minds, check out how right-wing extremists are using it these days. An example is Resistance Records, the world's largest purveyor of "hate-core" music.[10] Its recording artists include the rock band RaHoWa—short for Racial Holy War—whose song *When America Goes Down* includes the lyrics "the color of our skin [will become] our uniform of war." Resistance also features Centurion and their song *Fourteen Words* (the fourteen words, as the CD jacket notes explain, are "We Must Secure the Existence of Our Race and a Future for White Children"). Nordic Thunder's *Born to Hate* is also big.

Resistance Records is owned by 67-year-old William Pierce, perhaps the leading neo-Nazi in the United States and head of the white-supremacist National Alliance. Pierce wrote *The Turner Diaries*, which may have inspired home-grown terrorist Timothy McVeigh. Pierce is keenly aware that chronic exposure to certain types of music can prompt perfectly compliant citizens to question the wisdom of governments and religions in arbitrating their lives. And this is what institutions have always feared most about music and art—not the degradation of our morals, as they claim, but the capacity of music and art to point to a reality that transcends the authority of any government or religion.

Critical Care-oling

Music's power can be uncanny. Sometimes it seems almost capable of raising the dead, or at least the moribund.

Consider the case of Gerry McGlinchey, a 66-year-old man who suffered a brain hemorrhage from diving into a swimming pool in September 1999 in Cyprus. After spending five weeks in a coma, he was flown home to University Hospital, Aintree, Lancashire, where he could only respond with "Yes" and "No" to questions. Things changed abruptly on December 21 when a volunteer choir visited the hospital to sing Christmas carols. When they sang "Hark! The Herald Angels Sing," McGlinchey suddenly chimed in as his relatives listened in amazement. Then, with gusto and word-perfect clarity, he sang his heart out with "God Rest Ye, Merry Gentlemen," "The First Noel," and "We Wish You a Merry Christmas."[11]

Around the same time, Shawn Culle, a 27-year-old schoolteacher, lay unconscious in Basildon General Hospital in Tilbury, Essex, as a result of meningitis. Then fifteen children from St. Mary's Primary School, where he was a teacher, arrived and sang Christmas carols to him. From the moment they started singing, Culle began twitching and kicking and tried to remove his endotracheal tube. The nurses started to weep. Soon after, he was taken off life support. He was discharged two weeks later and made a full recovery.[12]

David Aldridge, Chair of Qualitative Research in Medicine, University of Witten Herdecke in Witten, Germany, reports other cases in which comatose patients in intensive care units have gained consciousness when a music therapist softly sings certain melodies to them.[13]

Lullabies

Mothers around the world sing lullabies to their babies, and research findings suggest the benefits can be dramatic, particularly for infants born prematurely.[14,15,16,17,18,19]

Before the thirty-fourth week of gestation, babies are not neurologically mature enough to master the "suck-swallow-breathe" rhythm required in feeding. Jayne M. Standley, director of the Center for Music Research at Florida State University in Tallahassee, and her colleagues invented a pressure-sensitive pacifier wired to a tape player that rewards hearty sucking by playing a lullaby recorded by a female performer.[20] When the baby ceased sucking, the lullaby shut off. The infants often mastered the skill in only minutes. Babies who were trained with the PAL (Pacifier Activated Lullaby) suckled 2.4 times faster than those not given the musical reinforcement. After only fifteen minutes of lullaby training, one preemie drained a full bottle of milk. Standley and her colleagues were amazed. "We thought it was our imagination—the response seemed too dramatic," she said. Field trials of a commercial variety of the musical pacifier are being spearheaded by Ohmed Medical in Columbia, Maryland.

Humming

Humming may also be good for the hummer. Anesthesiologists at Stockholm's famed Karolinska Institute have found that when people hum the oscillating sound waves reverberate through the sinus cavities that surround the nose and the eyes. These vibrations have a cleansing effect on the sinuses by clearing them of secretions and promoting air flow between the sinuses. Their research suggests that humming might be helpful in preventing or treating the sinus stuffiness of common colds and sinusitis.[21]

The sinuses are major producers of nitric oxide (NO), a gas that is made by a variety of plant and animal cells. NO is a small, reactive, and highly soluble molecule that passes easily through cell membranes and acts as a biological signal. In mammals, NO helps maintain blood pressure by dilating blood vessels, stimulates the immune system to kill invaders, and helps control penile erection (Viagra works by blocking an enzyme that metabolizes NO). NO also affects signaling between neurons in the brain and probably contributes to the formation of memories.[22] When the Karolinska researchers examined the level of NO in the paranasal sinuses of healthy individuals, they found that it increased fifteen-fold during humming compared with quiet breathing.[23]

Do dedicated hummers have better memories than nonhummers? Do they have a lower incidence of colds and sinus infections and do they throw them off more quickly? Are some sounds more effective than others when hummed? Does humming improve men's sex lives by churning out more nitric acid? These questions beg to be investigated, and any young researcher wanting to get his career humming might consider them.

Perhaps the most-chanted sound in the world is *om*, the sacred sound connected with Indian meditative traditions. In addition, sacred Gregorian and other chants have arisen for centuries from monasteries scattered throughout Europe. Chanting and humming in these traditions are not done to improve one's sinuses or any other aspect of physical health, of course, but as spiritual exercises and paths to the divine.[24]

And yet, immersion in one's own sonic vibrations *does* have healing effects. UCLA researchers found that if hospitalized schizophrenics hummed an *mmmm* sound, they experienced around a 60 percent reduction in auditory hallucinations.[25,26] Clinical reports abound in which angry, stressed-out, and chronically depressed people found inner balance and repose through humming, chanting, and toning.[27] Even physical symptoms can recede. When Marilyn Utz of Santa Monica, California, came home from work one day with a splitting sinus headache, she decided to forego pain medications in favor of toning. As she repeatedly emitted a long *ouuu* sound, she could feel her voice vibrate through her entire head. As she continued, her sinuses opened up and began to drain. She lapsed into quiet meditation and soon her headache disappeared.[28,29]

Purring

The soothing effect of lullabies and humming may be prefigured in how other species respond to gentle sounds. Take cats, for example. Scientists at North Carolina's Fauna Communication Research Institute have found that the purring of many felines—house cats, pumas, ocelots, servals, cheetahs, and caracals—falls within frequencies between 20 and 50 hertz (cycles per second).[30] It is known that when human bones are exposed to frequencies in this range, they tend to grow and become stronger and denser. Thus, scientists at Fauna believe cats may purr because it helps their bones and tissue to heal and grow stronger, perhaps helping explain why cats are considered to have "nine lives." Dr. Elizabeth von Muggenthaler, president of the institute, says, "We are starting to solve a 3,000-year-old mystery as to why cats purr. The next phase will be to explain the mechanics of the process."

Some people aren't convinced that purring helps cats recover from trauma. They point out that dogs don't purr, yet they also recover from falls at an impressive rate. In another survey done at Animal Medical Center, 80 of 81 dogs who fell from one to six stories survived.[31] So purring can't be the whole story behind cats' nine lives.

Dr. David Purdue, an expert in metabolic bone disease at Hull University in England, says that if purring does prevent dissolution of calcium and the weakening of cats' bones, it might be possible to devise a treatment using their purring to help strengthen osteoporotic bones in the elderly.[32] Does this sort of therapy already exist? Do elders who adore having purring cats continually nestled on their laps have a lower incidence of osteoporosis and hip fractures than their catless friends the same age?

Deep Music

Nearly two millennia ago, Gregory of Nyssa said, "If the arrangement of the whole is some kind of a musical harmony . . . in human nature, the whole music of the universe can be discerned."[33] Whereas Gregory saw music in the macrocosm, an increasing number of scientists see evidence of music in the microcosm—including even human DNA. As physician-researcher Lewis Thomas put it, "We are a spectacular, splendid manifestation of life. We have language. . . . We have affection. We have genes for usefulness. . . . And finally, and perhaps best of all, we have music."[34] Let's examine how pioneers in science have taken seriously the ancient idea that an innate musicality exists in our genes.

Susumo Ohno. "S. Ohno has cracked a new genetic code. [When this] 58-year-old geneticist . . . sets the genes to music—or music to genes—some strange and wonderful things occur. To wit: The SARS oncogene, a malignant gene first discovered in chickens, causes cancer in humans as well. When Ohno translated the gene into music, it sounded very much like Chopin's Funeral March. An enzyme called phosphoglycerate kinase, which breaks down glucose . . . in the body revealed itself to Ohno as a lullaby."[35] Science writer William R. Corliss thus describes the work of the late Susumo Ohno, a distinguished scientist at the Beckman Research Institute of the City of Hope National Medical Center, Duarte, California.

Ohno was the first scientist who, beginning in the 1980s, began to explore the musicality of the structure of genes by assigning musical notes to them according to their molecular weights. His goal was to discover a basic pattern—a melody?—that governs all life. His work triggered an outpouring of similar investigations into the intrinsic musicality of a variety of natural structures.

When I first discovered Professor Ohno's work with "genetic music" during the early 1990s, I wrote him and expressed my admiration for his work. He kindly sent me a tape of the music, performed by his wife Midori, a professional musician. The music was enchanting, as was the idea that I might be listening to music actually encoded in human DNA.

A few weeks later I was invited to give a lecture at a conference attended by a great many people with AIDS. At that time the treatment of AIDS was woefully inadequate. AIDS patients often had grotesque images of their bodies as infected, rotting, deteriorating death traps beyond hope of healing. I decided to play Professor Ohno's DNA music for the AIDS patients in order to give them, I hoped, a different image of their bodies. After the audience entered a meditative silence, the music began. One of the musical passages was indistinguishable from Chopin, another from Bach, another from Handel. Some of the music was lively, some sonorous, but all was beautiful. Soon people began to weep. When the music ended, they requested that it be replayed. By the end of this mini-concert everyone in the audience had begun to imagine their body in a different way, and there were few dry eyes.

Linda Long. Other scientists built on Ohno's pioneering work and carried it further. Among them is Linda Long, a biochemist, professional musician, composer, and research fellow in complementary medicine at Exeter University in England. Long is equally at home in herbal medicine, homeopathy, and music therapy, and her work linking music and biology has been funded by the National Endowment for Science, Technology, and the Arts.

Using X-ray crystallography, Long defines the three-dimensional positions of the amino acids in a particular protein molecule. This data is filtered and then mapped onto musical parameters such as pitch and amplitude. There is no arbitrary assignment of musical notes in this process. Protein helixes emerge as arpeggios; other structures take on additional musical forms. Long's work is a way of not just visualizing a protein's structural features, but hearing them too.

Most people aren't molecular biologists, so they don't respond to the complex visual models and data sets scientists use to describe the body's protein molecules. But humans have a keen ear for musical patterns, and music is not limited by words or logic. Thus Long's work has opened an acoustic door to the arcane world of molecular biology, through which nonscientists and even children and the visually impaired can enter. All that's required is the ability to appreciate a good tune.

Headed to England? Long's work is featured in "Listen to Your Body," a touch-screen interactive exhibit at Explore-at-Bristol, Bristol's new hands-on science center. Visitors can transform the shapes of their body's proteins into strings of melodies and follow a musical

trail through the human body. For information go to www.at-bristol.
org.uk.

Long also has an interest in herbal medicine, and has translated
proteins from a variety of medicinal plants into music. You can listen
to samples of the plant- and human-derived musical sequences, or
obtain a CD of them, via Dr. Long's Web site www.molecularmusic.
com.

Susan Alexjander. I have long been a fan of the work of musician
Susan Alexjander.[36] Working with University of California cell biologist David Deamer, she exposed sections of human DNA to infrared
light and determined the distinctive frequencies for each DNA molecule. Alexjander and Deamer then converted the ratios of light frequencies into ratios of sound. The result was haunting, beautiful
music with microtonal pitch changes, much like music we associate
with India and the Middle East.

Alexjander is cautious about what her DNA music means. Why
does it produce such strong reactions from people? She says, "Perhaps on a very deep level the body recognizes itself—hears something familiar in the music. It's a theory. I don't know."[37] But the artist
in all the explorers of the intersection of music and molecules knows.
They sense that their discoveries have revealed another world—not
the material, dead stuff of classical science, but something harmo-
nious, melodic, profound, and beautiful.

Alexjander's DNA music is available on CD from Science and the
Arts, P. O. Box 428, Aptos, CA 95010, or www.oursounduniverse.com.

Mary Anne Clark. Mary Anne Clark, a professor of molecular biology at Texas Wesleyan University in Fort Worth, also got hooked on
music and molecules.[38] Here is her description of her experience:[39]

> I . . . love to walk into the music building, which on my campus
> is next door to the science building. Through the doors of the

practice rooms, I can hear fragments of 1000 years of written music. . . . I think that if somehow I could walk into a living cell, I would hear something similar. . . . Every generation of cells in every living organism plays the genetic score of its species. However, while the history of music as we know it goes back some 1000 years, the history of genetic music is at least 3.8 billion years in the making.

Clark's work can be accessed at http://mitpress2.mit.edu/e-journals/Leonardo/isast/articles/lifemusic.html.

The Music of Geometry

Fractals—from the Latin *frangere*, "break"—are geometric shapes that look the same under any level of magnification. In fractal patterns, each structure is prefigured in every other. Examine a piece of a fractal and you get a copy of the entire structure. Fractals are ubiquitous and include most of the objects we encounter in daily life. A mountain and the rocks that make it up are fractal. So is a tree, its branches, twigs, leaves, veins, roots, and rootlets. Clouds, meandering rivers and coastlines, the timing of our heartbeats, the falling of snowflakes, and the distribution of galaxies in space are fractal. When fractals are translated mathematically onto computer screens, strangely psychedelic images appear, often of breathtaking beauty. As BBC science editor David Whitehouse says, "Fractals . . . have become a symbol of the profound mystery of numbers and the strangeness of order emerging from chaos."[40]

Could music be hiding in fractals? When British composer Phil Thompson translated fractals into music, he was "slightly scared" when he listened to the result. "What was coming out of the loudspeakers was not noise, it was recognisable music."[41] This doesn't surprise Ian Stewart, professor of mathematics at Warwick University and coauthor of *The Collapse of Chaos: Discovering Simplicity in a Complex*

World.[42] He observes, "Music has a certain structure, which our minds seem to like. You need theme and variation. By coincidence, or perhaps not, the mathematics of fractals is just like that."[43] People have responded enthusiastically to "musimatician" Thompson's music. When excerpts from his CD "Organised Chaos" were played on BBC Radio 4 in 1997, there was an unprecedented switchboard response. Thompson's fractal music is available through http:// artists.mp3s.com/artists/54/organised_chaos.html.

Whitehouse suspects that we respond to fractal music because of our species' history. He states, "Throughout our evolution we have been surrounded by fractals in the form of the noise of a waterfall, the rustle of undergrowth and the sounds of our own bodies . . . Perhaps that explains the sense of recognition we feel when we listen to fractal music?"[44]

The field of fractal music is thriving; there are more than 75,000 Internet listings under this category. Alternative therapists Aleia N. O'Reilly, Robert J. McCarter, and Steve D'Annunzio have produced a stellar video, "LightTones: A Journey of Color, Music, and Fractal Imagery," available through www.LittleHummingbird.com. Musician Patricia Mason offers a variety of fractal compositions at http:// users1.ee.net/pmason/music2.html.

Music in Nature

I travel a lot and sometimes have trouble sleeping in hotels. For years I have carried with me a gadget that plays a continual tape recording of a lively mountain stream. The musical sound of flowing water conjures images of happy moments spent trekking in mountains, backpacking, and fly fishing with Barbara and friends. This is the most effective sleep aid I have ever discovered.

Jim Nollman is a naturalist and author who is fascinated by the music nature makes.[45] He once met a man on the upper Kings River in the Sierra Nevada who told him that certain streams hold every song ever sung. Although Nollman considers this an exaggeration, he began to study the aesthetics of stream song. "The width and depth of a stream, its rate of flow, and its angle of descent mostly determine [a stream's] musical potential," he says. "Large roaring streams are too noisy to be musical. Lax-flowing streams are too quiet. . . . [T]he most musical streams vary between two and six feet in width and often lie just above or below alpine meadows where the land is sufficiently canted to produce small falls. Mere drips falling down a stairway of ledges into deep pools usually provide the most pleasing timbres." Nollman finds that pleasant tones seem to emerge best just following dusk, when the air gets cool and vapor collects in the bottoms of canyons, enhancing the bass tones that fall silent during the heat of the day.

The most musical stream Nollman ever encountered is Wright Stream, a few miles southwest of Mount Whitney in California. The first evening he camped there he listened to a deep baritone emerging from the stream singing the "Toreador Song." He was so enchanted he decided to stay another night. The second evening he heard a singer who sounded like Elvis crooning a ballad he'd never heard before. (Those Elvis impersonators are everywhere.)

Nollman says of his experience, "I conclude that some of humanity's most ancient tunes were learned by our distant ancestors while camped on the slopes above musical streams. Music that they heard rising from the falling waters they attributed to fairies—water spirits—who hid in the rock cavities by day and emerged at dusk to start their all-night songfests. No doubt, one of the listeners learned the tune and taught it to the rest of the tribe. The people may have named certain streams after individual fairies. And when their progeny revisited the same stream a hundred years later, the tribe's songline map of the mountains cued them to listen to the same fairy singing a tune they then knew by heart."[46]

Musical sounds also crop up in some of the driest places on the planet, such as the Sahara and at least thirty other desert sites around the world.[47] The earliest reports of "the singing desert" are from ninth-century Chinese literature. Marco Polo was captivated by these noises during his trek across the Gobi desert in the thirteenth century, attributing them to the spirits of the desert. The sounds vary; singing, humming, booming, roaring, drumming, trumpetlike, and other resonances have been described. Research suggests they are triggered by sand particles avalanching down the sides of the dunes. "The cascading sound behaves like the membrane of a loudspeaker moving at a frequency that generates audible sound," says researcher Bruno Andreotti of the University of Paris.[48] The internal structure of the dune may also play a part. The hard, compacted area just under the surface may resonate like the soundbox of a musical instrument, amplifying the frequencies set up by the sliding sand.

Calming the Inner Surgeon

Even though many studies show that music can calm patients undergoing surgery, what about the surgeons operating on them? Psychologists Karen Allen and Jim Blascovich, of the State University of New York at Buffalo, were the first researchers to study this question.[49] Their studies were published in 1994 in the *Journal of the American Medical Association.* Their experiment involved fifty male surgeon volunteers, ranging from thirty-one to sixty-one years old (mean age, 52). All the surgeons described themselves as music enthusiasts who listened regularly to music during surgery. The surgeons were examined in a soundproof laboratory under three conditions—while listening to a piece of music they selected, while listening to music selected by the experimenters (Pachelbel's Canon in D), and while listening to no music. During each condition they were asked to perform a mental task that is known to be emotionally stressful—counting backward rapidly out loud by subtracting 13s, 23s, 27s, 43s, or 47s serially from a five-digit number. During all sessions their pulse rate, systolic and diastolic blood pressures, and skin conductance were measured, all of which indicate levels of stress in autonomic activity. The speed and accuracy with which they accomplished their mental task were also measured under the three conditions. The findings: Pulse rate and blood pressure were significantly less, and speed and accuracy of task performance were significantly better while the surgeons were listening to music they selected themselves than while listening to the experimenter-selected music, or to no music at all. The 50 surgeons chose 50 different pieces of music, all instrumental—forty-six classical, two jazz, and two Irish folk. The type of music did not matter; self-selection was the key.

This study points out a recurring finding: In music's effects on the body, there are no absolutes. The music that soothes one individual may drive another to distraction.

The researchers concluded, "In 1889, Nietzsche wrote, 'Without music life would be a mistake.'[50] Over a century later, our data prompt us to ponder if, without music, surgery would be a mistake."

Sick Brains Respond

Surgeons presumably have normal brains. Can music calm people whose brains are abnormal?

Dr. Ardash Kumar, associate professor in the Department of Psychiatry and Behavioral Sciences of the University of Miami School of Medicine, and his colleagues performed the first experiment examining the impact of music on patients with Alzheimer's disease.[51] Using twenty male inpatients diagnosed with this problem at the Miami Veterans Administration Medical Center, they exposed them to thirty- to forty-minute sessions of music therapy five times per week for four weeks.

The sessions included singing led by the music therapists playing keyboard and guitar. The patients were invited not only to sing but also to play musical instruments and handheld flat drums using their hands or mallets. The therapists accommodated the patients' choices of songs, which were quite varied. In one group, one patient liked only Broadway or big band tunes, another preferred opera, another liked spirituals, one wanted country and western songs, another Cuban folk music. Patients were also encouraged to improvise tunes and create musical sounds on xylophones. Every attempt was made to keep them involved with musicmaking throughout the sessions.

As the program progressed, impressive behavioral changes began to take place in the patients. They demonstrated greater calm and well-being. Their ability to sing and learn new songs and to follow rhythm and tempo improved. Their interaction with their fellow patients and the therapists increased.

Blood samples were obtained before initiating the music therapy program, immediately at the end of the four-week program, and six weeks after the program ended. They found that melatonin concentration in the blood increased significantly after the music therapy program and continued to increase even further at six-weeks follow-up. Norepinephrine and epinephrine levels also increased significantly after four weeks of music therapy, but returned to pretherapy levels by six weeks after the music was discontinued. Levels of prolactin and serotonin remained unchanged from baseline during the study and during the follow-up period.

"Music therapy might be a safer and more effective alternative to many psychotropic medications," said Dr. Kumar.[52] "Like meditation and yoga, it can help us maintain our hormonal and emotional balance, even during periods of stress or disease."

The researchers were intrigued that melatonin, which is considered the messenger molecule of the pineal gland, was the hormone most affected by the music therapy. "Even in ancient times," they noted, "the pineal gland was considered the 'seat of the soul,' a concept borrowed from ancient Greece and elaborated by Descartes. Mystics and yogis in India have described the spiritual and beneficial effects one experiences through yoga and meditation as being mediated by stimulation of the pineal gland. Music therapy may therefore be considered among the important resources for enhancing melatonin release via pineal gland stimulation and for unlocking and restoring the expression of emotional connections with our deeper self, whether in a state of health or disease."[53]

Girls, Boys, and Music

I took piano lessons when I was growing up, an experience I treasure in retrospect. Back then, however, I was ambivalent, because music lessons seemed mainly a "girl thing." Girls just seemed to catch on quicker than us thick-headed, ham-fisted boys. So I am not surprised that research has recently shown that female birds learn music more quickly as well.

In most bird species in temperate climates, only the males sing, but among northern cardinals both males and females become singers. Yale University biologist Ayako Yamaguchi raised twenty-six hatchlings in separate chambers and exposed them to recordings of at least forty songs of adult cardinals.[54] Both females and males began to learn songs at about three weeks following hatching. Although both the girls and boys eventually learned about the same number of songs, the females did it in one-third the time. They required only about fifty days to complete their repertoire, after which their sensitive learning period shut down, while the males' period stretched to around 190 days.

Why the slower learning in males? In the wild, a long, drawn-out learning phase means that males would keep on learning new songs even after they leave their parents' nests and venture into new territory. Yamaguchi suggests that this would help the males pick up the song accents of their new neighborhoods and hold their own in the singing duels by which males declare and defend their territories.

As Harvard psychiatrist Gregg D. Jacobs describes in his book *The Ancestral Mind*, birdsong contains remarkable parallels with human music.[55] Birds use the same rhythmic variations and combinations of notes as we do, they recognize and memorize musical patterns, and they share songs and pass them along from one generation to the next. Some birds have mastered musical instruments. For example, as part of his courtship ritual the male palm cockatoo of northern Australia selects a twig from a tree, breaks it, then shapes it into a drumstick. Then, holding it with his foot, he beats on a hollow log.[56]

Not only are humans drawn to birdsong, birds are also attracted to the music we make.[57,58] Jacobs describes an interaction between Mozart and a starling, a species skilled in creating and imitating songs.[59] While Mozart was composing a piano concerto in G major, the starling began singing part of it. "In one of his notebooks," says Jacobs, "Mozart recorded the starling's interpretation of the final movement of the piece. Although many of the starling's notes were the same as the composer's, the bird also improvised, and quite 'beautifully,' as Mozart noted."

Gray Matter

Does listening to classical music make infants and children smarter? In 1993, UC-Irvine physicist Gordon Shaw and cognitive development expert and former concert cellist Frances Rauscher played the first ten minutes of Mozart's Sonata for Two Pianos in D Major, K.448, to a group of college students.[60] There was an increase of around eight or nine points in the students' IQ scores as assessed by spatial-temporal reasoning—the ability to visualize something in space that unfolds over time, such as estimating how a piece of paper will look unfolded. Although the increase in IQ lasted only about ten minutes, the "Mozart effect" was born. The media caught on, and almost overnight, parents across the United States were wondering if they should expose their children to Mozart or other classical music in order to increase their intelligence.

However, the picture quickly became cloudier. Although Shaw, Rauscher, and Ky replicated and extended the original findings,[61] other researchers could find no effect at all.[62,63]

The leading proponent of the Mozart effect is musician and educator Don Campbell, author of the bestselling book *The Mozart Effect*.[64] His enthusiasm for the effects of Mozart's music is based not only on the implications of the studies of Shaw, Rauscher, and Ky, but also on the discoveries of physician Alfred Tomatis.[65] Tomatis was the first researcher to develop a technique using music to stimulate the rich interconnections between the ear and the nervous system to enhance human development and behavior.

Although there is no consensus in the academic music community on the validity and significance of the Mozart effect, it has been widely embraced by the public. While it is true that much work remains to be done in assessing the impact of classical and other types of music on early childhood development, researchers in this field, as in all areas of complementary and alternative medicine, need elbow room to explore boundary issues without being shouted down.

Music, Against All Odds

Why do we make music? Perhaps because we must, no matter how difficult it may be to do so. As Flaubert wrote in *Madame Bovary*, "We long to make music that will melt the stars."[66]

The famous violinist Itzhak Perlman was stricken with polio as a child and walks with the aid of crutches and leg braces.[67] When he comes onto the stage he has to make an enormous effort—putting his crutches down on the floor, unlocking his braces, tucking his feet just so, reaching for his violin before he can begin to play.

At a concert on November 18, 1995, things did not go smoothly for Perlman. After only a few bars, a violin string snapped with the sound of gunfire. The audience realized that the concert would have to pause for him to laboriously and painfully adjust his braces, pick up his crutches, walk off stage, and repair the string or find another instrument. Instead, Perlman paused, closed his eyes, and signaled the conductor to continue playing from where he had left off.

As Rabbi Jack Reimer, who was present that night and related this account, said, "And he played with such passion and such power and such purity as [we] had never heard before. Of course, anyone knows that it is impossible to play a symphonic work with just three strings.

I know that, and you know that, but that night Itzhak Perlman refused to know that. You could see him modulating, changing, recomposing the piece in his head. At one point, it sounded like he was de-tuning the strings to get new sounds from them that they had never made before."[68]

When he finished, the audience was stunned, and rose to its feet, applauded, and cheered. Reimer continues, "He smiled, wiped the sweat from his brow, raised his bow to quiet us, and then he said, not boastfully, but in a quiet, pensive, reverent tone, 'You know, sometimes it is the artist's task to find out how much music you can still make with what you have left.'

"So," Reimer concluded, "perhaps our task in this shaky, fast-changing, bewildering world in which we live is to make music, at first with all that we have, and then, when that is no longer possible, to make music with what we have left."

Countering Violence

In ancient Greece, music was considered an art of the Muses, the nine goddesses who presided over literature and the arts and sciences. For the Greeks, music could delight and charm, but it could also spellbind and bewitch. We have largely forgotten that music has two sides—that it can transport us to the majestic heights of human thought and feeling or nudge us toward the brink of hell, as when the Nazis used Wagner's music as a tool to implement their goals.

The power of music to influence the fate of nations was acknowledged in Greece and elsewhere. "In India, Greece, and China," writes musicologist Jill Purce, "music represented the order of the universe. No Chinese emperor would come to power without making sure that music was in order, because he knew that if music wasn't in order there would be chaos and revolution."[69]

How will *we* use music? It does not dishonor great music to ask this question. And if we fail to ask, music will use *us*, as the German nation discovered too late during World War II. Composer-conductor

Leonard Bernstein realized that music could be used as a force for good. He said, "This will be our reply to violence: to make music more intensely, more beautifully, more devotedly than ever before."[70]

Can music moderate the violence of our post-9/11 world? In our current shock-and-awe strategy toward terrorism, could music be used as a vehicle for delivering the awe without the shock? These questions are worth asking, because throughout history music has been capable of making governments and institutions tremble, as we have seen. Music remains one of the most effective bridges between cultures that exists. Unlike the machinations of diplomacy, there is little artifice in many kinds of music. An example is jazz, that quintessentially American invention that sprang from the soul of black musicians in New Orleans in the late nineteenth century. The legendary pianist Charles Mingus knew the honesty of great jazz. "In my music," he said, "I'm trying to play the truth of what I am."[71] Perhaps jazz's straight-ahead honesty is why some of our most effective cultural ambassadors have been jazz musicians.

But bridging cultures is not enough. If we are to survive and flourish on this planet, we shall also have to stem the violent ways we have behaved toward the earth and its creatures. A factor that might unite us with other living things is music. Scientists have identified music in the DNA and genes of a huge variety of living things, from viruses to humans.[72,73,74,75] Essayist Verlyn Klinkenborg describes how music binds together all of life:

> [S]cientists [have mapped] out an affinity for music in a wide array of species. This is not just a chronicle of grunts, squeaks and warbles. . . . [These findings] suggest that . . . our love of music is no less instinctual than it is in animals and that our remarkable skill as music-makers gives us no grounds for self-exaltation. . . . Seen for what we are, co-inhabitants of a slim wet planet, co-evolved under the same strains, the same harmonies, collaborators in a shared environment, how could the resemblance be less than they are?[76]

It is not surprising that the earth is alive with music, because the universe is too. In 2003, astronomers at Cambridge University in England reported their discovery of sound waves emerging from the Perseus galaxy cluster, which is 250 million light-years from Earth.[77,78] This cluster of galaxies is heated by a massive black hole that is one billion times heavier than our sun. This super-heating is believed to generate the sound waves, which are B-flat in pitch, fifty-seven octaves lower than the tones of a concert piano, far below the range of human hearing.

Andrew Fabian, one of the astronomers involved, believes this sort of music is widespread. "We expect every cluster group of galaxies has its own note," he says, "and lots of tunes are being played throughout the universe."[79]

The idea of "the music of the spheres" has been around since Pythagoras, but has been dismissed by scientists as nonsense. Now the idea is confirmed.

Given the unimaginable number of galaxies in the universe, a continuous pulsing, throbbing symphony is playing out there. One day, when we record and amplify all the individual notes, what will the music sound like?

I'm betting on Bach.

Risk

A ship in port is safe, but that's not what ships are for.

—GRACE MURRAY HOPPER, REAR ADMIRAL,
UNITED STATES NAVY

All writers engage in rituals to get their creative juices flowing. Sometimes these practices are exalted, such as listening to inspiring music, and sometimes they are mundane. My writing rituals fall into the latter category.

When I get up in the morning to write, before going to my computer I put on my hiking boots. They don't come from the Abercrombie & Fitch fashion catalog. They're the real thing—heavy-duty leather, over the ankle, scuffed and scarred. The point? Writers need to take chances, go to insecure places, put something on the line. I associate the boots with risk-taking and close calls when I have worn them on hiking and camping trips atop the Continental Divide. I have a superstition that if I wear my boots while writing, risk-taking may seep into the writing process. And with my boots on I feel better equipped to engage in the perpetual task of the writer, which is to comfort the afflicted and afflict the comfortable.

In addition, I have a blizzard of quotations taped to my printer that encourage me. One is from actor Robert Strauss: "It's a little like wrestling a gorilla. You don't quit when *you're* tired, you quit when the *gorilla* is tired." And an anonymous aphorism advises me, "Don't worry about what people think; they don't do it that often." I also have a collection of totems and fetishes on my desk, all symbols of boldness and risk-taking. A miniature Native American tomahawk dangles from my computer, a reminder that warriorship is essential to good writing. Close by sits my favorite compass (I own six), which reminds me to stay on track. Also on my desk is a paperweight in the form of a turquoise ceremonial axe, a gift from anthropologist-author Lyall Watson, who found it in the mountains nearby. He traces its origins to the savage Aztec society that lay to the south of Santa Fe, where I live. Watson, who knows about these things, assured me that if I kept it on my desk it would add fire to my scribblings. And on one wall hangs a cluster of talismans from various traditions, to retard the hexes and curses that could come my way from people I am sure to offend if I do my job well.

From my boots up, I've structured my writing environment to remind me to take risks. I know, I know: all this could be interpreted as pathological behavior—unconscious hostility and unfulfilled aggression, or old boys and their toys. But as Freud said, sometimes a cigar is just a cigar.

Why this flirtation with risk-taking? I believe the urge to take risks is innate, inscribed in bone and blood and genes, and that when we completely avoid risk, we sabotage our greatest potential.

Our culture's myths affirm this view. The Grail legend, which mythologist Joseph Campbell proclaimed the most influential Western myth, is all about risk. In it, King Arthur and his knights are at table, about to feast, but Arthur will not permit the festivities to begin until an adventure has occurred. Suddenly, the Holy Grail appears and hovers above the table, but it is draped and cannot be fully seen. Then it vanishes. Gawain, Arthur's nephew, solemnly proposes that all the knights embark on a quest for the Grail, so that it can be glimpsed in its fullness. The knights agree—but, realizing that it would be cowardly to go in a group, each resolves to make the journey alone, to enter the forest at its darkest point, where there is no light, no path, and no guide—the epitome of risk.

The Grail quest is a symbolic journey toward psychological awakening and enlightenment. It champions and celebrates risk, and it teaches us that a quest without risk is not genuine, but an exercise in self-indulgence. When artists face a blank canvas, when writers stare at a blank sheet of paper or an empty computer screen, they confront the age-old questions of whether to play it safe or leap into the unknown.

I feel connected with the Arthurian legends. Three years ago, Barbara and I journeyed to Tintagel Head, a cape on the coast of Cornwall in southwestern England. According to legend, Tintagel was the birthplace of King Arthur. This is a land of rocky, plunging coastlines that are smothered with cloud and mist, where ferocious winds howl and the surf booms—the perfect birthplace for someone whose legend would teach the Western world about the transformative power of risk.

Arthur's Britain taught me another lesson. I was born during a dark moment in history—the early days of World War II prior to America's entry into the conflict, when Hitler was trying to break England's back by attacking London from the air. I had long been curious about what happened in London the day I was born. So, on a recent visit there, I rummaged through archives that recorded the daily death toll during the blitz. I discovered that my birth date was bloody—a day on which many Londoners lost their lives to the Nazi bombs.

I had always imagined that the psychological shock of the blitz would be devastating. I was surprised to discover that during the air raids, admissions to mental hospitals in London, as well as the suicide rate, dropped. A survey of fifty British psychologists showed that even patients who were mentally disturbed prior to the bombing improved during the blitz, and that the people who showed the greatest improvement were those who were assigned the most dangerous tasks, such as fighting fires and rescuing victims. Similar patterns were found elsewhere and in other illnesses. For example, it was predicted that the heart-attack rate would increase during the war because of psychological stress, but in France it actually decreased.[1,2,3]

Taking risks, then, is good not only for writers and artists; it can also be valuable for people's health. From the way we pathologize risk, you would not think this is the case. We require people who are engaged in high-risk occupations, such as commercial ocean fishing, to pay higher insurance premiums. We consider participants in risky sports, such as bungee jumping and hang gliding, as semideranged. We have become so intolerant of risky behavior that a movement has sprung up in education that, according to anthropologist Stephan Schwartz, "increasingly considers being a boy a diseased state."[4] Thus, we have created diagnostic categories for rambunctious, risk-loving boys, and have taken to Ritalinizing boyish behavior out of existence. We prefer undisruptive kids who grow up to be mellow adults who are properly horrified by unsafe behavior in all its forms.

Black Magic

The idea of health risk is inseparable from the theory of probability, which John von Neumann, perhaps the greatest mathematician of the twentieth century, called "black magic." Probability seems magical because of a paradox: Although it can predict with incredible precision the overall result of a large number of events, the individual events themselves are *un*predictable. As novelist Arthur Koestler put it, "[In probability,] we are faced with *a large number of uncertainties producing a certainty.*"[5]

Statisticians, for example, can forecast the total number of dog bites in New York City in a given year, but they are unable to predict whether the dog approaching you in Central Park is going to take a bite out of your ankle. Physicists can foretell the half-life of a radioactive substance, which is the time it takes for half its atoms to disintegrate, but not when a particular atom in the substance will decay. Casino owners can estimate the percentage of people who will win and lose at their gambling tables, but they don't know whether you are going to lose or break the bank on your next throw of the dice.

Because statistics can seem impenetrable or even threatening, most people consider them largely useless in making decisions about how to lead their lives. This attitude can have lethal effects. Following the terrorist attacks and the crashes of four passenger jets on September 11, 2001, droves of people abandoned flying and chose to drive instead. This fear of flying triggered an increased death toll as a result of the overcrowding of America's roads and the increase in car crashes. During the final three months of 2001, an extra 353 car-crash deaths occurred, compared with the average number of auto fatalities for the same months from 1996 through 2000. These extra deaths exceeded the 266 lives lost on the four doomed planes. The fatalities did not surprise statisticians, but the public still seems to be in denial of them. Although flying remains the safest mode of transportation in the United States, air travel is still down and auto travel remains up.[6]

We ignore the messages of probability even when they are comforting. If we responded rationally, we would conclude that we live in the safest nation that has ever existed, and we would worry less. Yet, we have taken to worrying more. As journalists Jane Spencer and Cynthia Crossen observe, we see danger lurking everywhere.[7] If scalding coffee from McDonald's doesn't get us, mad cow disease, SARS, anthrax, or West Nile virus will. We cringe when the Homeland Security department ups the color-coded terrorism alert, although our chance of being bagged by a terrorist is remote. We worry about being blown out of the sky by someone with a bomb in his shoe, even though only one such threat has ever been detected. Parents fret that their children will be killed by unsafe toys or poisoned by salmonella in their McFood—all these worries in spite of the fact that our average life span is 60 percent longer than in 1900. As politicians have learned, we are easy to scare, but impossible to unscare. It seems as if we *want* to be terrified, like teenagers who flock to horror movies, and not even the reliability of statistics can comfort us.

Skydiving and Cancer

Physicians sometimes say things they would never want their patients to hear, such as the choices they would make if they were sick. An oncologist I know is adamant that if he develops terminal cancer he would not undergo chemotherapy and irradiation, which he prescribes for his patients on a daily basis. He says he would move to Hawaii instead, which is his favorite place on earth, and lay in a plentiful supply of his favorite Scotch whiskey and liberal doses of morphine for pain.

I once asked a psychologist friend of mine, who counsels cancer patients, what he would do if he developed cancer.

"I'd take up skydiving," he said without hesitation.

"Why?" I asked.

"The idea of skydiving freaks me out," he replied. "That's why it would be the perfect cancer therapy for me."

He explained that people who experience spontaneous remission from cancer often do so after taking up habits that are totally foreign to their temperament, and which frequently involve considerable physical risk.

Evidence suggests he may be correct. An active immune system is essential in rejecting cancer and infections, and it can be stimulated by risky behavior. Researchers Douglas Granger and Alan Booth, of Penn State University, and David R. Johnson, of the University of Nebraska, have shown that men who are moderately aggressive have stronger immune systems than men who are perfectly behaved.[8] They found that men who have been in occasional fights or been in trouble with the law, either as young people or adults, have immune systems that respond more rapidly and intensely to infection and cancer. It makes sense, say the researchers, because aggressive, risky behavior throughout history has been associated with gaining access to food, resources, and territory, as well as battling predators and protecting mates and offspring. These behaviors also lead to trauma and infected wounds. Therefore, those individuals who have more robust immune systems would be better survivors, and immune competence, aggression, and risk-taking would tend to become genetically linked and passed down through succeeding generations. Risk, therefore, and the stress that comes with it are not always bad.

An experiment in risk-taking took place on a huge scale in the second half of the twentieth century, when millions of American women began entering the work force. Many observers (almost all male) predicted doom. They said that leaving one's sheltered role as homemaker, wife, and mother would expose women to enormous stress and put them at risk for health problems. Evidence suggests that the opposite is true.[9] In a study in San Antonio involving 422 Anglo and 623 Mexican-American working women and housewives, the working women had superior profiles on three indicators of cardiovascular health: higher levels of high-density lipoprotein or "good" cholesterol, lower levels of low-density or "bad" cholesterol, and lower levels of triglycerides.[10] Another study of married, middle-aged American working women found they had better health than did housewives, provided they had positive attitudes toward their jobs.[11] And a University of Michigan survey found that women who held three, four, or five roles did not report greater conflict or stress in their lives than women with only one or two roles.[12]

Risk-Taking Americans

If risk-taking makes people healthier, you might think Americans would be the healthiest people on earth. From the Pilgrims and the pioneers who settled America, to the entrepreneurs and venture capitalists of our day, we are known as a nation of risk-takers. We like this image of ourselves, and have always celebrated it in literature, music, and film. Historical evidence suggests, however, that this image is inflated. For example, the mortality rate on the wagon trains that went west, though significant, was not nearly as high as was once thought. Wagon-train pioneers were far more likely to be killed by accidents with the firearms they brought along than by hostile Indians.[13]

Historians have also called into question the risk the pioneers faced once they got where they were going. One study found that 70 percent of the westbound immigrants who left towns in New England and New York returned to the comforts of their former homes within only a few years.[14] What prompted their return was generally not the dangers of the frontier but "the wretched loneliness and almost total lack of excitement in their lives."[15] In short, they were bored.

Compared to modern-day Americans, however, our predecessors were profound risk-takers. Ralph Keyes is the author of *Chancing It: Why We Take Risks,* one of the best books ever written on this subject. During the twentieth century, we witnessed the gradual development of what he calls the American Way of Risk: "a stimulating, exciting, even heart-thumping form of excitement with no danger, stakes, or risk of any kind except the loss of quarters" in video arcades, virtual reality booths, theme parks, sports stadiums, NASCAR race tracks, and movies.[16] Innocent pursuits? Not according to Keyes. Take computer games. Their danger for young players, he says, is that the world they represent is phony, because there is no real danger and therefore no consequences. Game-players may get sweaty palms, but they never get dirty or bloody. And because no risk or courage is called for, there is never any genuine emotional catharsis. This is why, says Keyes, computer games become boring and must be replaced every six months to a year, and why America's theme parks continually install new rides that promise more novelty, titillation, and thrills.

Yet, Americans hunger for authentic risk and will go out of their way to experience it. When a fatality occurs on a ride in an amusement park, the operators know that when the ride re-opens the waiting lines for it will be longer than ever. National park supervisors know that reports of bear attacks in a particular area will make that area more popular. Following the release of the movie *Deliverance,* dozens of drownings occurred on Georgia's turbulent Chattooga River, where the movie was filmed, as people flocked to experience it.[17]

When computer games, theme parks, and movies minimize what genuine risk really is, they can pose threats to health. Consider Outward Bound, which champions what the company calls "expeditionary learning" in wilderness settings. The image that is projected, says Keyes, is that of an outdoor encounter group. But over the years, over a dozen participants have died in these courses.[18] In exploring Outward Bound's on-line marketing information (www.outwardbound .com), I could find no explicit mention of the risk of death.[19] The company does acknowledge that its instructors are trained in CPR, but does not explain why they need to be, and there is a refund policy for individuals who may be injured. But nowhere can one find an unambiguous caution to parents that their kid could die while participating in the course.

I am a fan of Outward Bound and applaud its efforts to introduce urban kids to wilderness, and I know that nearly all kids fortunate enough to participate in its programs come back enriched, wiser, and unharmed. But every time we gloss over genuine risk, we misrepresent the real world to our children and to ourselves. As a result, the world becomes increasingly distorted. Eventually all forms of mayhem, even including war, can seem little more than an exercise in virtual reality, in which nobody really gets hurt.

Acceptable Risk

When I first began practicing internal medicine, I was baffled by patients who said, "Cancer is the best thing that has ever happened to me." Although the disease varied, the message was the same: an illness and a brush with death had enriched and transformed their lives. At the time, I was impatient with these comments. I was trained to stamp out disease, not honor it. People will stop at nothing, I thought, to rationalize their predicaments and put a good face on a bad situation. Years later, I see it differently. Although I do not recommend serious illness to anyone, these individuals nonetheless underwent a profound reshaping of their life's values and meanings by experiencing risk, and they believed the risk was worth it.

What is an acceptable risk?

It depends on who we are—our make-up, our personality, our temperament. What feels risky to one person may seem boring to another. With risk, one size does not fit all.

In his book, Ralph Keyes distinguishes two kinds of risk, which he calls Level I and Level II.[20] Level I is what most people imagine risk-taking to be—dangerous, highly exciting activities that usually don't last very long. Level I risk-takers tend to be aggressive, extroverted, restless individuals who value action and excitement, and for whom boredom and routine are anathema.

In contrast, Level II risk is usually not dramatic or physically dangerous, is longer lasting, and is more challenging to the psyche than to the body. Level II risk-takers tend toward introversion, conformity, and patience. They are even-tempered, calm individuals who value attention to detail, security, control, and predictability.

Level I risk-takers would be more likely to prefer motorcycles over bicycles, downhill over cross-country skiing, and high-contact sports over golf. Level I individuals are more likely to choose careers such as combat soldiering, politics, law enforcement, entertainment, or journalism. Level II persons prefer careers such as archaeology, library science, computer programming, novel writing, dentistry, medicine, pharmacy, or academia.

A classic Level I risk-taker is former governor Gary Johnson of New Mexico. During his second term in office, he went to the edge of political respectability by condemning America's war on drugs as a complete failure, and by championing the legalization of drugs in the United States. These stances were considered by many to be political suicide, and they were unpopular even in his own state. But the governor thrived on challenges and controversy. While in office he continued his devotion to extreme sports. Once he nearly drowned and had to be rescued while kayaking a stretch of white water on the upper

Rio Grande. He participated in the Boston Marathon and the Hawaii Ironman triathlon, and after stepping down as governor, he climbed to the top of Mt. Everest in 2003.

But Levels I and II are generalizations. No one is a pure Level I or Level II risk-taker; we have elements of both, and the types of risk we prefer may shift at different periods of our life, as they should. Yet the levels perspective is valuable because it helps us individualize the notion of risk, and helps us avoid the fallacy that one person's idea of risk is valid for everyone.

To be genuine, says Keyes, "Risks must be authentic, genuinely daring for the risk taker."[21] But that does not mean risks have to be fear-filled and physically dangerous. Genuine risk must push us outside our comfort zone. For writers and artists, as I have mentioned, this means venturing into unfamiliar dimensions where failure, embarrassment, and rejection lurk. Writing is a classic Level II risk. It would be boring to a Level I risk-taker, who would prefer almost anything to typing for hours on a keyboard.

Genuine risk should not be sociopathic or illegal, and can frequently substitute for behaviors that are. Keyes reports that thieves, drug dealers, and users he has known have found that alternative forms of Level I risk-taking have satisfied their craving for excitement. Among these activities have been mountaineering, scuba diving, and skydiving.[22] High-risk teens have also successfully switched to activities such as joining volunteer fire-fighting squads, the Marines, or, in some instances, going to a military academy. Other kids' lives have been transformed by wilderness experiences, or taking up outdoor sports such as fly-fishing or hunting. Peace Corps activities, which offer young people the opportunity to live and work in foreign lands beyond the comforts of home, have fulfilled the hunger for risk for thousands. So, too, has AmeriCorps, the domestic program which since 1993 has offered more than 200,000 individuals the opportunity to be "in service to America."

During my years as an internist, I have seen hundreds of eager teens volunteering as "candy stripers" throughout the hospital. The services they provide are so essential that I can't imagine how some hospitals could run without them. Candy stripers are exposed to the blood and gore of emergency rooms, which can more than gratify their yearning for excitement. The tasks they are assigned, such as ferrying blood from the blood bank to a hemorrhaging patient in the ER, often make an impression that remains with them for the rest of their lives.

Hospitals are fabulous places for experiencing risk, because things there happen so unpredictably, as I learned as a first-year medical student. I was enrolled at Southwestern Medical School in Dallas, and spent time at Parkland Memorial Hospital, the medical school's main teaching hospital. One dull November day in 1963, I was amazed at the chaos I encountered at Parkland as I was returning from lunch. Policemen and armed guards were everywhere. I asked a security guard what was going on, and he said, "The President has been shot." I was standing near a pay telephone in the ER. The phone had been commandeered by Robert Pierpoint, the nationally known CBS News commentator, who was traveling with the presidential party on President John F. Kennedy's visit to Dallas. I was wearing a short white jacket, the sign of a first-year medical student. I suppose I appeared reliable, because Pierpoint introduced himself to me and said urgently, "Will you help me? Guard this phone with your life." He handed me the phone, which was connected to CBS headquarters in New York City. For more than an hour, Pierpoint and I worked as a team. While he dashed into the hospital to the President's trauma room, I relayed observations to the office in New York. That experience is seared into my memory.

Donating part of one's own body, such as blood, appeals to thousands of individuals as a mild form of risk-taking with considerable social value.[23] One psychiatrist[24] has suggested that another medically useful form of thrill-seeking is to donate other parts of one's body— organs such as bone marrow, a kidney, or a part of one's liver. If you think this is an outrageous suggestion, you are probably a Level II risk-taker. Many Level I individuals would be excited at the chance.

After all, they risk more than a kidney each time they sky-dive, bungee-jump, or ski off a precipice.

An increasing number of young people are finding fulfillment in academic programs such as environmental science, marine biology, or climatology, which often combine intellectual excitement with physical risk. Research in these areas can carry them to the ends of the earth to hostile geographic locations. They find satisfaction in knowing that their findings on global warming or environmental degradation may have life-and-death consequences for the entire planet.

Why Risk?

Why do we take risks? Hypotheses abound. Freud considered risk-taking to be a veiled expression of Thanatos, the death wish. Some biologists believe that aggressiveness and risk-taking are genetically determined. Others say that the sensation-seekers become hooked on the fluxes of their own brain chemicals, which create a pleasant high during physically dangerous experiences. Some scientists maintain that hormones such as testosterone push people toward risk-taking, especially in adolescent males. Others say it works the other way round: Hormones such as testosterone don't *cause* risk-taking and aggression, but they increase *as a result of* violent activity—the chicken-or-egg problem. Recent evidence from brain scans suggests that teenagers take more risks than adults because they can't foresee the consequences of their actions. Some researchers believe this indicates the immaturity of juvenile brains and is a reason why the death penalty should be abolished for juvenile offenders under the age of eighteen.[25] Some psychologists insist that cultural, social, and psychological forces are the main initiators of risk-taking behavior.[26] A great many researchers hedge their bets and opt for a combination of genetic, hormonal, psychological, and cultural factors.[27]

Many biologists believe risk-taking by males is a ritual that makes them more attractive to a prospective mate.[28] How else can one explain male behaviors, such as running with the bulls at Pamplona, staged in front of thousands of shrieking females, in which hundreds of men run down the city's narrow streets within inches of the horns of running bulls, risking goring and death?

Yet explanations of risk-taking that rely on blind genetic urges and the surges of neurotransmitters, I feel, leave something out. Consider the high-altitude, hot-air balloonist Steve Fossett. On the surface, Fossett seemed to be bent on self-destruction in a series of failures and crashes before he succeeded in circumnavigating the planet on his sixth attempt in July 2002.[29] Prior to this achievement he raced cars, sailed catamarans, and climbed mountains. In 1985 he swam the English Channel from France to England; in 1992 he completed Alaska's Iditarod Dogsled Race. He set eight official records for ocean-sailing, including the Yokohama-to-San Francisco record.

Level I risk-takers are often viewed as out-of-control, testosterone-charged males who should know better. If they wind up a motionless mass at the bottom of a canyon or the ocean, they deserve it. Yet Fossett is no hotheaded idiot, and the fact that he is still alive speaks volumes about successful Level I risk-takers. He is a highly intelligent planner who obsesses over details and leaves nothing to chance. He serves on the Board of Trustees of Washington University in St. Louis; is a fellow of the Royal Geographical Society and the Explorers Club; and is devoted to making his adventures accessible to kids online.

One of Fossett's heroes is the Norwegian polar explorer Fridtjof Nansen (1861–1930). Nansen was such a consummate planner that in his many polar explorations he never lost a member of his team. Nansen was also a scientist and humanitarian, was awarded the Nobel Peace Prize, and was Norway's delegate to the League of Nations.

Level I risk-takers are not always careful, of course, and their lives frequently end tragically because they refused to wear a motorcycle helmet or a life jacket—a mistake which a Fossett or a Nansen would never make. Others, such as Christa McAuliffe, a gung ho school-teacher from Concord, N.H., who died in the 1986 *Challenger* disaster—her "ultimate field trip"—pay with their lives not because of their own mistakes but because others on their support team take short cuts.[30]

Regardless of why they do it, we owe Level I risk-takers a lot. Our lives have been immeasurably enriched by high-riskers past and present, people such as Lewis and Clark, Sacajawea, Daniel Boone, Sally Ride, Sir Edmund Hillary, John Wesley Powell, Amelia Earhart, Marco Polo, Christopher Columbus, Jedediah Smith, and Susan Butcher. They have defined for us the limits of human possibility. Without individuals such as these, humankind would stagnate. They return from their adventures with insights they share with those who stay behind, and their legends become crucibles into which the timid can dip vicariously.

Religion

The most popular risk-reduction program in history is religion— trusting God, Goddess, Allah, or some other version of the Almighty to make a difference in one's life, including one's health. There is a lot to say for this point of view. For the first time in history, empirical evidence suggests that, on average, people who follow a religious or spiritual path—it doesn't seem to matter which—live significantly longer than people who do not, and have a lower incidence of most major diseases.[31,32,33] In addition, several controlled studies indicate that intercessory prayer and healing intentions can improve health outcomes in those toward whom these efforts are directed, even when the recipient is unaware of them,[34,35] and that participation in prayer and meditation benefits the pray-er or meditator as well.[36,37,38] But caution is required. Religion sometimes increases health risks. Just because something is holy doesn't mean it's healthy.

Throughout human history, including today, religion has often been used as a pretext for war and the slaughter of millions of humans, most often noncombatants. And during the Middle Ages, condemnation as a heretic by religious authorities proved lethal to thousands of innocents.

Spiritual rituals have often posed health risks. During the eighteenth and nineteenth centuries, smallpox decimated the Native American tribes of North America. These epidemics are believed to have been worsened by the ritual of the sweat lodge, in which participants sit unclothed in a steamy, sealed enclosure. As medical historian R. S. Bray observes, "This has generally been considered an excellent method of disseminating smallpox . . ."[39]

Sun-gazing, an ancient religious ritual, has caused solar retinopathy and irreversible visual loss.[40]

Death from heat stroke has always been a problem during pilgrimages to Mecca.[41] In Sweden, where sunshine is in short supply much of the year, Muslim women who cover themselves from head to toe are at risk of vitamin D deficiency from too little sun exposure.[42] Muslims who perform industrial work during the fasting period of Ramadan have collapsed due to dehydration and circulatory failure.[43]

One out of every twelve people on earth live in the basin of India's Ganges River or its tributaries, whose waters are sacred to millions of Hindus. Tragically, the river has become a 1,400 mile-long conduit for raw sewage, human and industrial waste, animal carcasses, and the partially cremated bodies of humans. At the holy city of Varanasi, the Ganges contains an astonishing 340,000 times the acceptable level of fecal coliform bacteria, and outbreaks of waterborne diseases such as hepatitis, cholera, typhoid, and amoebic dysentery are common along its entire course. Although they are bathing in a veritable soup of pathogens, some 60,000 devotees take their holy dip each day at Varanasi alone. Many drink the water, believing it to be pure and invigorating. Drinking and bathing in the waters of "Mother Ganges" constitutes perhaps the greatest health risk, for more people, than any other religious ritual on earth.[44]

A recent study from Duke University Medical Center revealed an increased risk of dying when illness strikes, if the individual experiences a sense of religious struggle. Mortality was highest among those who wondered if God had abandoned or was punishing them, and in those who questioned God's love or who believed the devil made the illness happen.[45]

In the 2001 Irish Young Scientist contest, three 14-year-old competitors examined the purity of holy water contained in the fonts of local churches in County Kildare. They came up with the project when one of the girls developed a rash on her forehead after blessing herself with holy water. They found tiny green worms in one font and large quantities of dirt in others. It wasn't the first time that young sleuths had exposed Ireland's holy waters as unclean. In 1998, student scientists from County Clare grew coliforms, staphylococci, yeast, and molds from local fonts. And in 1999 some Dublin churches removed their fonts altogether from the vestibules when they discovered that drug addicts were using them to rinse their syringes.[46]

Risk-taking can lead to accidents, illness, and death, but, as we have seen, it can also make us healthier. Risk is a paradox, which has been defined as truth standing upside down to attract attention.

Do risk and safety really contradict each other? Many ancient philosophers said no. They maintained that opposites were actually in cahoots with each other. Oppositional relationships were fundamental, they said, a kind of glue that held the world together. As the ancient Greek sage Hermes Trismegistus allegedly said, "By the friendship of contraries, and the blending of things unlike, the fire of heaven has been changed into light, which is shed on all below . . ."[47] And Heraclitus: "The harmony of the world arises from opposites held in tension, as in the lyre and the bow."[48] Research such as that of Granger, Booth, and Johnson, as we saw, is revealing the paradoxical health benefits of risk-taking, and is a humbling example of how modern science is playing catch-up with this millennia-old point of view.

This ancient wisdom still lives. It is present in our competing biological urges to play it safe and also to take risks. This paradox is our birthright—and a reminder that our obsession with creating a risk-free existence, from the nursery to the crematorium, is folly.

I often wonder how much healthier we would be if we honored the value of both risk and security, health and illness—acknowledging that, as Thoreau put it, "'Tis healthy to be sick sometimes."[49] The goal in this recognition would not be utilitarian, such as living a decade or so longer, but to allow the flowering of a psychospiritual peace in our lives, the consolation of knowing we are going with the grain of the world instead of against it.

Simone Weil, France's great essayist and spiritual seeker, understood how contraries connect. She wrote, "The prisoners whose cells adjoin communicate with each other by knocking on the wall. The wall is the thing which separates them but is also their means of communication. It is the same with us and God. Every separation is a link."[50]

The final word goes to America's eminent social commentator, Dolly Parton. Though more prosaic than Weil, she makes the same point: "If you want the rainbow, you gotta put up with the rain."[51]

8

Plants

Never go to a doctor whose office plants have died.

—ERMA BOMBECK

From the way we talk, you'd think we humans were plants. We grow like "weeds" in childhood, "blossom" as we mature, and go to "seed" as we age. New ideas get "planted" in our minds, where they "germinate," "take root," "flower," or "wither." We "weed" out bad ideas, "cultivate" good will, and "reap" what we "sow." We raise "seed" money for new businesses, "farm" out projects to others, and join "grass-roots" movements. We collect "kernels" of wisdom, follow decision "trees," and "branch out" in our activities. We may go out on a "limb" and get lost in a "jungle" of detail. Someone who doesn't see the big picture is a "blooming" idiot who can't see the "forest" for the "trees." Surgeons perform "implants" and "transplants," and physicians do "stem" cell research. We "leaf" through books and turn over a new "leaf" in our behavior. Political parties search for presidential "timber" and we elect presidents named "Bush." We liken our entire trajectory through life to plants. As Dennis Stillings, of Hawaii's Archaeus Project, states,[1] "We grow as a plant in the womb, starting as a seed, absorbing nourishment directly through our umbilical 'root,' well-watered, and located within the mother (*mater* = mother = matter), the timeless symbol of the earth itself. In the end, for all our frantic activity, we are again 'planted' and the grasses and trees have their way with us."

These expressions point to our "green consciousness"—the fundamental psychospiritual connections we share with the plant world. These bonds are really not surprising, because at a deep level we know that without plants, humans could not exist.

During my residency in internal medicine, several of my physician colleagues and I were at a party. The atmosphere was especially celebratory because we were nearing the end of some of the most difficult years of our training. Suddenly Matthew, a close friend since medical school days, collapsed into a chair with a groan. He was pale and sweaty and could not stand because of agonizing pain in his left foot. Matt had come down with an acute attack of gout, which had plagued him all his adult life. Acute gout is one of the most intense varieties of pain known to humankind. The site of Matt's affliction was classic: the great toe of one foot. In old woodcuts and drawings, the pain of gout is often represented as a small dragon or demon with its claws and fangs dug into one's foot. "Please take me to the emergency room!" he pleaded. I half-carried him to the car, and we sped to the hospital where we both worked. By the time we arrived at the ER the pain was truly horrific; Matt was grimacing and could hardly speak. He knew from past episodes what relieved them: an intravenous injection of colchicine, a substance derived from the plant *Colchicum autumnale.* Colchicine is one of the most fabulous plant medicines in history—a specific therapy for a specific problem—and has been used for centuries. Following Matt's instructions, I started an IV and filled a syringe with the clear solution and began the injection. Then magic happened. Before half the injection was in, he bounded to his feet with a smile and announced, "The pain is completely gone. Let's get back to the party!" This event was one my of my most vivid lessons in the extraordinary healing power of ordinary things, and to this day seems nearly miraculous.

Listening to Plants

One of the most popular herbs in the United States is *Ginkgo biloba*, which comes from the leaves of the ginkgo tree.[2] The main reason people consume ginkgo is to perk up their cognitive powers and memory.[3] Ginkgo has been around for 200 million years and is considered by botanists to be something of a living fossil. Is it merely coincidental that a tree, whose genetic memory reaches back 2 million centuries, is being used to treat problems with our own memory? It's as if the ginkgo tree is saying to us, "Hey, I've got this memory thing down pat. Want some help?" I'm suggesting a level of communication between plants and animals that may help explain why we use specific plants for certain maladies.

Consider, for example, how folk healers and plants interact on the island of Madagascar, as reported by biologist Lyall Watson. It has been more than a hundred million years since Madagascar split off from Africa, drifted into the Indian Ocean, and became isolated.[4] The runaway island carried a rich cargo of plants and animals, many of which continued to evolve and are found nowhere else. Humans, however, are rather new there, arriving only in the last two thousand years. These African and Asian immigrants confronted nearly fifteen thousand species of flowering plants, 90 percent of which they were totally unfamiliar with from their previous habitats. Yet in a mere hundred generations they managed to sort through this huge inventory of exotic plants, so that today they have an impressive array of useful herbal remedies for sale in any market. How did they do it? There simply hasn't been time to test every strange plant, and determine which part of the plant, in which season, and from which species, works best—and whether it should be eaten whole, boiled, dried, or fresh. As Watson succinctly puts it, they must have had help.

And the help, it seems, comes from the plants themselves. When Watson asked a local healer how they know that an extract from the leaves of a local flowering plant, picked in the spring, is good for a condition they call "milky blood," he always gets the same answer. "Oh, it's easy," they say, "we ask the plants."[5]

It may sound absurd to Westerners, but that's exactly what these healers do. They enter the forest while thinking about a particular patient and wander around with an open mind. Eventually a plant catches the healer's attention and declares itself the proper remedy. Watson was skeptical about this process until he discovered that the above-mentioned condition the local healers call "milky blood" is leukemia, which literally means "white blood" because of the color that is often imparted by an excessively high white blood cell count. And the plant the healers chose for use is a lovely pink flower called the Madagascar periwinkle, from which a major pharmaceutical company extracts the drugs vincristine and vinblastine, used to treat certain types of leukemia.

Native healers use a variety of ways to listen to medicinal plants. Botanist and artist Kat Harrison, who has roamed the world talking with native healers, has tried some of these methods herself. Her studies took her to the upper Amazon near Iquitos, Peru, where she worked with mestizo people of Indian and Spanish lineage. "It was suggested to me that I do their way of instant bioassay of a plant," she relates. "You would take a few leaves and crumble them and rub them on your face and forehead. Then lie down in the hammock or sit in the forest with your eyes closed and become very receptive, suspend judgment, be clear, and find whatever occurs. It is the unbidden information that's actually valued the most. That which we don't lead, that which we don't direct."[6]

The natives even used Harrison as their plant medium, their surrogate listener. When she first arrived, she was quickly attracted to a plant called *labios de la sirena*, siren's lips. Her hosts considered this plant thereafter as her ally, and suggested that she put some of it under her pillow at night. When she awoke the next morning, six people were waiting to hear her dreams. "I had amazing dreams," she reports, "really the most beautiful, consistently positive, long, and totally memorable dreams I've ever had in my life, and I'm a good dreamer . . . I would like to dream like that every night."[7]

The methods used by native healers in identifying medicinal plants is a stark contrast to the industrial, workmanlike screening processes employed by modern labs. For instance, each year the National Cancer Institute (NCI) receives around 4,000 samples from all over the world, representing some 2,000 species of plants, herbs, microbes, and marine specimens.[8] Researchers test organic and water extracts from each sample against the AIDS virus and sixty human cancer cell lines. If a specimen selectively kills its target, it then goes through a purification process to isolate the chemical constituents responsible. Only then can a compound start the journey toward clinical trials and potential approval as a drug. Since 1986, only about 1 or 2 percent of the 70,000 extracts screened by the NCI have turned out to be selective killers, and many of these proved too toxic for human use. In fact, only two successful drugs were produced between 1960 and 1980, both used against cancer—Taxol, derived originally from the Pacific yew tree, *Taxus brevifolia,* and a modified version of camptothecin, from the Chinese Tree of Joy, *Camptotheca acuminata.*[9]

These mass screening methods are slow, mind-numbing, and expensive. You'd think the drug screeners would try speeding things up by bringing in native healers who can hear the plants talk—and indeed they are. Author Kenny Ausubel, in his inspiring book *Restoring the Earth: Visionary Solutions from the Bioneers,* reports that the National Institutes of Health has begun working closely with herbal healers in many countries to identify new drugs, and that drug giant Bristol-Myers Squibb has made deals with native healers in Asia to look for native plants.[10]

We'd *better* listen up. As noted Harvard biologist E. O. Wilson points out, "Few are aware of how much we already depend on wild organisms for medicine. In the United States a quarter of all prescriptions dispensed by pharmacies are substances extracted from plants. Another 13 percent come from microorganisms and three percent more from animals, for a total of over 40 percent that are organism-derived."[11]

Hope for Doctors

How do indigenous healers know what the plants are saying to them? The trick is learning how to listen without censoring or getting in the way. This requirement puts us Western physicians at a serious disadvantage. We don't even listen to people, much less plants. According to a 1999 survey published in the *Journal of the American Medical Association*, a patient has only twenty-three seconds on average to state his or her concerns during a visit to a doctor before being interrupted.[12]

I believe, however, that we physicians can learn to listen to plants. I got a hint of what the listening process is like while obtaining an undergraduate degree in pharmacy prior to going to medical school. My favorite course was pharmacognosy, the study of medicinal plants. The pharmacognosy lab doubled as a museum, its walls lined with desiccated specimens of medicinal plants from all over the world. Ginkgo was on the shelf, as was colchicine, and a huge jar of the dried leaves of marijuana, *Cannabis sativa*. Although the marijuana was unguarded, no one ever stole it. I often wondered why. The reason, I'm convinced, was what the plants were saying to us. Entering the lab was like venturing into the workspace of a medieval herbalist. All the herbal specimens, including marijuana, had a hallowed aura about them, and I swear that on occasion—in the quiet moments—I could hear the old plants speak. Stealing marijuana or any other specimen would have been almost unthinkable, the equivalent of purloining a sacred relic.

Human-to-Plant Communication

When we speak of people having green thumbs, we acknowledge that they have a special gift for relating to plants. We also recognize the opposite potential—those who have black thumbs. The basic idea is

that some people have healthful effects on the living things that surround them, while other individuals have toxic influences. When we
select a physician, it is important to distinguish between the two. As
the late humorist Erma Bombeck said in the epigraph of this chapter,
"Never go to a doctor whose office plants have died."[13]

Currently, we select straight-A college students in biology, chem-
istry, and math to enter medical school. But what if there were other
indicators of talent, such as one's influence on living things such as
plants? Could we possibly use the responses of plants to identify natural healers, those individuals in whose presence living things flourish? In the past few years, laboratory experiments have come close to
doing just that.

In one particular study, psychologist Bernard Grad, of Canada's
McGill University, investigated whether or not mental depression
might produce a negative effect on the growth of plants.[14] Grad theo-
rized that if plants were watered with water that had been held by
depressed people, they would grow more slowly than if watered with
water held by people in an upbeat mood. A controlled experiment
was devised using a man known to have a green thumb and two
patients in a psychiatric hospital—a woman with a depressive neuro-
sis and a man with a psychotic depression.

Each person held a sealed bottle between his or her hands for
thirty minutes, which was then used to water barley seeds. The green-
thumb man was in a confident, positive mood at the time he held his
solution, and his seeds grew faster than those of the others and the
controls. Unexpectedly, the normally depressed, neurotic woman
responded to the experiment with a brighter mood, asking relevant
questions and showing great interest. She cradled her bottle of water
in her lap as a mother might hold a child. Her seeds also grew faster
than those of the controls. The man with the psychotic depression
was agitated and depressed at the time he held his solution; his seeds
grew slower than the controls. Grad's study suggested that (1) human
thoughts and emotions might influence living systems, positively and
negatively, and (2) physical objects might mediate these influences.

Grad performed three similar experiments, but instead of using psychiatric patients he used a healer. The outcome was significant in all three runs of the experiment: The seeds watered with a solution the healer had held, in an attempt to impart healing power to it, germinated and grew better than seeds in the control group.

Grad extended his experiments to animals, and found similar effects in wound healing and tumor growth.

Encouraged by his work, researchers all over the world have performed additional studies documenting the effects of one's mental state and intentions on a variety of living systems—growth rates of bacteria, plants, and cells; the activity of key biochemical reactions; and the rate of mutations within cells.[15,16]

These experiments show clearly that some people have healing influences on living things, and others do not. They also show that individuals can work things both ways: they can either increase or *decrease* the healthiness of living systems, depending on their mental intentions.

The implications for healing, and for how we select young doctors, are profound. A talent for healing—and its opposite—clearly exists, as all indigenous cultures have recognized. Our goal should be to select those with natural talent, just as we select gifted students in mathematics, music, athletics, and most other fields. And one way of identifying them is to ask the plants.

People have sensed that plants are sacred since the dawn of human history. As writer Robert Lee Hotz says, "The earliest physical token of humanity's spiritual yearnings are traces of ancient pollen from hyacinth and hollyhock flowers—the remains of what many scholars believe was a garland placed by a mourner in a Neanderthal grave more than 44,000 years ago."[17]

Perhaps it is the sacredness we sense in plants that accounts for their ability to summon us to greater health when we are in their presence. Consider a famous 1976 study by psychologists Ellen Langer and Judith Rodin.[18] They gave one group of nursing home residents potted plants to take care of, while offering suggestions on doing more for themselves rather than letting the staff take all the responsibility. A second group, matched with the first for degree of ill health and disability, received the usual nursing home treatment, along with assurances that the staff would handle all decisions and responsibilities. By three weeks, the potted plant group showed significant improvement in health and the amount of activity engaged in. The results were even more dramatic after eighteen months. The death rate of the potted-plant group was only 50 percent that of the other group.

This classic study is always interpreted as an example of the health-enhancing effects of taking charge and assuming responsibility. But what called these factors forth and set them in motion? Perhaps the potted plants, by their mere presence, enabled the nursing home residents to listen to the admonitions of the nursing staff in a new way. Or perhaps the elderly residents weren't listening to the staff at all, but to the plants.

Take Two Aspirin

How alike are plants and people?

Florists commonly tell their customers to put an aspirin tablet in a vase of cut flowers to make the blooms stay fresh longer. Biochemist Ralph A. Backhaus and his colleagues at Arizona State University in Tempe have turned up evidence supporting the florists' advice.[19] They have discovered that aspirin works in both humans and plants in the same situation—when they have been cut, scraped, or bruised.

In animals, aspirin blocks the production of prostaglandins, which are fatty acids that initiate an inflammatory response and constrict blood vessels. In plants, aspirin blocks the production of jasmonic acid, which causes leaf-eating bugs to produce chemicals that give them indigestion. The biochemical steps that are inhibited by aspirin in both plants and animals are surprisingly similar.

Jasmonic acid not only helps plants fight off bugs, it hastens aging in plants as well. Botanists suggest that premature aging in injured plants may be an attempt by the plant to generate seeds before dying. In one study, wild radish seedlings that had one of their four leaves eaten by caterpillars went on to produce 60 percent more seeds than unnibbled controls.[20] So the florists are right on target: aspirin really does cause freshly cut blooms to "stay young" by shutting down age-promoting jasmonic acid.

None of the scientists involved in this research suggest that aspirin actually relieves pain in plants, because they don't believe plants sense pain. However, might the response of injured plants to aspirin, which has perhaps relieved more pain in humans than any other substance in history, be a clue that plants might feel pain to some degree? If this sounds outrageous, we have only to recall that in the nineteenth century most scientists believed that *animals* did not feel pain, but this view is no longer held. Could we be wrong about plants too? I know, I know: it is philosophically reckless to attribute human feelings to inanimate entities. Professional philosophers have a name for this lapse in logic; they call it the "pathetic fallacy," although they have never adequately explained why it is either pathetic or fallacious to believe that feelings extend beyond the human domain.

The answers we give to the question of plant feelings have real consequences for how we live our lives. One of the most common reasons people choose vegetarianism is that they believe plants don't feel and that animals do, and they do not wish to cause pain in what they eat. Our self-image is tied up with this choice. As Cardinal John Henry Newman (1801–1890) put it, "It is almost a definition of a gentleman to say that he is one who never inflicts pain."[21] But in view of the above considerations, we might reevaluate this vegetarian defense. Could it be that vegetarianism seems more acceptable because we simply aren't listening to the plants? If we took seriously the implications of those biochemical processes in plants, which sound as if they are geared to relieve pain, would we be so cavalier about eating them? Would we continue to behead cabbage plants, amputate asparagus, thresh wheat, boil onions, flay apples, crack nuts, press garlic, chop carrots, drown (soak) beans, squeeze oranges, roast potatoes, skin bananas and cremate (flambé) them, and blend all sorts fruits and vegetables to smithereens?

I'm not advocating abandoning vegetarianism. But if we took seriously the possibility of pain perception in plants, perhaps we'd eat them with a bit more gratitude, and also with the realization that the plants will have their turn to eat us when we are eventually "planted."

Plant-to-Animal Transplants

One of the criteria for determining biological similarity is whether or not tissue from one living organism can be successfully transplanted to another. If the transplant takes, the donor and recipient are said to be "compatible." It has been assumed that plants and animals are so dissimilar that transplants between the two are not possible. But in 1995 a research team headed by Xavier Lozoya at Mexico's National Medical Center successfully transplanted plant tissue into animals for the first time in history.[22] They call these studies *inter-regni* experiments—"among kingdoms."

Lozoya and his team transplanted plant tissue from *Mimosa tenuiflora* into the subcutaneous tissue of rats and performed microscopic studies of the grafted areas at thirty, sixty, and one hundred twenty days following transplantation. Contrary to conventional predictions, the plant grafts survived. Following an initial inflammatory response, a fibrous capsule formed around the transplanted material and by the fourth month, capillaries and small blood vessels gradually formed inside the grafts. This suggested to the researchers that perhaps there are unknown mechanisms nourishing plant cells, and that metabolites produced by the plant grafts might be transported into the bloodstream of the host animal. The plant material was eventually removed from the rats and was re-grown outside their bodies, proving that it had remained viable all the while. These findings, said the researchers, suggest that plant grafts might serve as a source of pharmacologically active compounds. Lozoya's experiments give an entirely new slant to "growing your own."

What Would Nature Do? Aping the Apes

Janine Benyus, a forester in Montana's majestic Bitterroot Valley, works with biomimicry, which she describes as "the conscious emulation of life's genius."[23,24] She suggests that before trying to solve a problem, we ask ourselves, "What would nature do here?"

Let's look again at the problem of how to identify medicinal plants in a tropical rain forest. One way to proceed is to ask Benyus's question, what would nature do here?

The answer took on new meaning for Michael Huffman, of Kyoto University, while he was watching a parasite-ridden, constipated chimpanzee called Chausiku in the Mahale Mountains of western Tanzania.[25] Huffman saw the chimp reach for the shoot of a noxious tree that chimps usually avoid, peel it, and eat its bitter pith. Within 24 hours, all of Chausiku's symptoms had vanished. It was the first time a scientist had seen a sick chimp select an unsavory plant known by humans to have medicinal properties, consume it, and then recover. Huffman looked on in awe, realizing that he may have been observing the origins of human botanical medicine. Since then, numerous examples of animal self-medication have been documented, helping to lay the foundation of the growing field of zoopharmacognosy.

In Borneo, tropical forest specialist Willie Smits spotted an orangutan clutch its head as if it suffered a headache, pluck a flower from a certain plant, and munch it. A short time later it went happily on its way. The next time Smits got a headache in the rainforest, he plucked and ate the same remedy, with the same result.

Huffman and a host of other researchers, inspired by the work of famous chimpanzee specialist Jane Goodall, have found that chimps swallow single, whole leaves from any of thirty-four different trees. The leaves emerge intact and undigested in the dung, with neatly defined, concertinalike folds. The chimps' leaf-swallowing habit peaks about two months after the beginning of the rainy season, which is also peak time for infection with a major intestinal parasite. Huffman has discovered that only sick chimps swallow the leaves. All the leaves, he finds, have bristles on their undersides. When examined, live worms are found caught among the hairs and folds of the defecated leaves. Huffman's "Velcro theory" is that the leaves pass through the intestine, snag the worms, and shuttle them out of the body.

Most self-medication in wild primates involves chemical rather than mechanical processes, however. For example, mountain gorillas in Uganda eat the bark of the dombeya tree as food, which is laced with natural antibiotics lethal to *E. coli* and other pathogens. The bitter pith that Huffman saw Chausiku eat is from the tree *Veronica amygdalina*, which has been found to contain compounds active against many of the organisms that cause malaria, dysentery, and schistosomiasis. The local WaTongwe people take the same plants for the same problems as the chimps, and they recover within the same time frame.

One of Huffman's key discoveries is that the pith the chimps eat contains around twenty compounds that have different levels of activity and exert different effects on intestinal parasites. "Some of the most bioactive compounds," he says, "act to paralyze the worm, inhibit movement, prevent egg laying. Other compounds are toxic [to the parasite]."

In modern medicine, we have opted for the magic bullet approach—the single-drug, single-action method of totally eradicating a pathogen. This promotes drug resistance, because the single mechanism stimulates the pathogen to develop a counter-strategy. In contrast, reports journalist Aisling Irwin, "Forest remedies rarely expunge the disease entirely; they just suppress it. The leaf-swallowing chimps still carry parasites, but in low, safe numbers. At the end of the rainy season, infections disappear naturally."[26]

Opponents of herbal medicine disagree with this approach, sometimes with good reason. In some diseases such as AIDS, the carrier state is dangerous and should be eliminated. On other points, however, the herb foes may be considerably off base. They don't get the herbal principle of multiple compounds acting mildly and synergistically. They assume that there is *one* key compound in the herb that can be isolated, synthesized, and used in pure form. Yet, zoopharmacognosy suggests that herbs may work because of the sheer variety of the sub-stances they contain, not because of any single compound.

Herbal medicine is like killing flies with lots of flyswatters, not nuking them with a single lethal weapon. Although some of the flies may survive the flyswatters, so, too, may the patient.

How did the chimp Huffman observed know which plant was the correct one? The chimp didn't go to a doctor for advice; he either knew intuitively which plants worked, or was taught by other chimps. But what is meant by "instinct"? And if he was taught by other chimps, how did they originally acquire this knowledge? By trial and error? Perhaps. My hunch, however, is that something primal is going on, something that transcends random experimentation—perhaps the sort of thing that still seems to occur when the native herbalists of Madagascar need help from plants. The herbs themselves get involved. They respond; they talk back.

Critics

We simply cannot understand the popularity of herbs without taking our green consciousness into consideration—which, suggests zoophar-macognosy, has been developing for a very long time.

Many critics of the use of herbal medicines do not trust the intra-psychic forces that bind us to the green world, and they want to do battle with them. They believe that the choices people make about the medicines they use should be based solely on controlled clinical trials, and they see America's fondness for green medicine as a dangerous antiscientific trend. Thus, William Jarvis,[27] of the National Council Against Health Fraud, has called the idea of whole-herb medicine "ideological pap," unsupported by scientific evidence. Proponents of herbal medicine, he charges, have "a love affair with nature that sees it only as benign or benevolent, without looking at the dangerous side." The most implacable foes of herbal medicine seem to believe that herbs—nature in the raw—can't be trusted; they must be tamed by isolating their active chemical compounds, synthesizing them, and marketing them as a pharmaceutical product available only by prescription. This point of view implies that reliable medicinal wisdom was absent before the appearance of randomized clinical trials around the middle of the twentieth century.

Critics of herbal medicine do not realize that humankind has been involved in a continuous, worldwide drug experiment for hundreds of thousands of years. This colossal experiment has been made up of untold numbers of single-case studies involving the use of herbs in every culture on earth. Every time an indigenous healer administered an herb to a sick individual, experience was gained and the knowledge got around. This ongoing planetary experiment dwarfs anything conceived by our National Institutes of Health and pharmaceutical companies. Yet the wisdom gained is too often disregarded, to our collective detriment.

The critics of herbs are correct about one thing, however: there are hazards to green medicine. Some herbal preparations are toxic, which would be foolish to ignore.[28] But the current debate about the dangers of herbs often becomes overheated and unbalanced, especially in view of the fact that each year the side effects of pharmaceuticals are responsible for the deaths of around 100,000 hospitalized Americans,[29] and that hospital care in general rates currently as the third major killer in the country, following heart disease and cancer.[30] Of course, the defects of conventional medicine do not justify shortcomings in the use of herbs or any other therapy, but they do suggest that critics often invoke a double standard where herbs are concerned.

A Little Respect?

I come from generations of farmers. Perhaps that's one reason I naturally respect the contributions plants make to human welfare, and why I recoil when I see medicinal plants treated disrespectfully by professionals, who you'd think would know better.

Consider the anticancer drug Taxol, which the National Cancer Institute recently touted as the biggest therapeutic breakthrough in cancer treatment of the past two decades.[31] Taxol was originally derived from the bark of the Pacific yew tree, *Taxus brevifolia,* as mentioned earlier. When the compound was initially discovered, six one-hundred-year-old yews had to be sacrificed to recover enough drug to treat a single patient. At this rate the tree would have become rapidly extinct in the Pacific Northwest. Because of the outcry of environmental groups, the pharmaceutical industry found ways of growing their own yews rather than cutting down wild ones, and of extracting the active ingredient from the yew's needles. The results have been spectacularly rewarding for drug giant Bristol-Myers Squibb. In 1996 alone, global sales of Taxol exceeded $800 million, lending additional meaning to "green" medicine.[32]

Here's how the drug company describes Taxol in the venerable *Physicians' Desk Reference* (PDR): [33]

Paclitaxel [Taxol's generic name] is a natural product with antitumor activity. The chemical name for paclitaxel is 5β, 20-Epoxy-$1,2\alpha$, $4,7\beta$, 10β, 13α-hexahydroxytax-11-en-9-one $4,10$-diacetate 2-benzoate 13-ester with ($2R$, $3S$)-N-benzoyl-3-phenylisoerine. . . . Paclitaxel is a white to off-white powder with the empirical formula $C_{47}H_{51}NO_{14}$ and a molecular weight of 853.9. It is high lipophilic, insoluble in water, and melts at around 216-$217°C$.

This is like describing *Mona Lisa* in terms of the chemical composition of the pigments Leonardo used. Aside from referring to Taxol as a "natural product," no mention is made of the Pacific yew tree in the company's entire four-page description, in spite of the fact that without the tree the drug would not exist. After yielding its precious medicine, the yew has been cast aside. It does not merit even a footnote of gratitude, an honorable mention, a sideways glance. You'd think that a company that reaps around $1 billion a year from a plant might pay it a bit more respect in print. No wonder Taxol causes wretched side effects—more than two pages of "Warnings" and "Adverse Reactions"—as if this is its way of protesting the insult.

Loving Herbs to Death

According to the World Health Organization, approximately 80 percent of the world's inhabitants rely on traditional plant-based medicines.[34] For centuries, harvesting these substances from the wild or from small homegrown gardens posed no problem, because people gathered or grew only what they needed. But as international interest in herbs has increased, demand is outstripping natural production for many herbs and the plants are in trouble. We may be loving some of them to death.

It has happened before. In the seventh century BCE, a band of Greek settlers from Thera founded the city of Cyrene, in modern-day Libya. They must have questioned the oracle's advice to settle there because the landscape was parched and the natives were unfriendly. But they soon discovered Cyrene's single asset—a species of giant fennel called silphium, which eventually made the colony rich. Although silphium was used as a condiment and cough suppressant, its effectiveness as a contraceptive was unparalleled. Soranus, the second-century Greek physician, wrote that the juice from a chickpea-sized portion, taken once a month, was enough to prevent pregnancy. Silphium, however, was maddeningly scarce, growing exclusively in North Africa along a thirty-mile strip of land near the city. It was finicky too: attempts to transplant it to Syria and Greece were a failure, to the delight of the Cyrenians. Prices rose quickly. By the beginning of the first century CE, silphium was more costly than silver by weight and had become the contraceptive of aristocrats. Three centuries later it was extinct.[35]

Many modern herbs, like silphium, are in trouble. Consider goldenseal, *Hydrastis canadensis,* which is used to treat infections and is one of the best-selling herbs in the world. Although this small woodland plant grows abundantly in moist hardwood forests around the world, large-scale collection combined with burgeoning timber harvests is making it increasingly difficult to find goldenseal in forests where it once was plentiful. The herb requires decades to reestablish itself, and current demand threatens to decimate the species.[36]

Ginseng may be hardest hit among the herbs that are in current high demand. It is an extremely slow-growing root, requiring a minimum of six years to mature, and only the fully mature plant has medicinal value. Although more than 90 percent of ginseng exported from the United States is cultivated, the poaching of wild ginseng has skyrocketed because it fetches $1,000 per kilo—more than three times as much as the cultivated.[37] American ginseng tops a recent list of endangered plants compiled by United Plant Savers, a group of concerned herbalists and conservationists based in Vermont. Goldenseal and wild yam, *Dioscorea villosa,* from which the anti-aging hormone DHEA is derived, occupy second and third place on the list. The Convention in Trade in Endangered Species has also begun to compile its own list of rare medicinal plants that require protection.[38] Journalist Nathaniel Mead suggests that the power of the market, which has threatened many species of herbs, may eventually prove to be their salvation. "As wild-harvested herbs become more scarce, quality is likely to decline while prices increase. . . . This makes cultivation increasingly profitable. And with appropriate growing techniques, the quality of organically grown herbs can meet and even surpass that of their wild counterparts. As a result, growing medicinal plants may become a booming business."[39] Yet it is a heartless approach, driving plants to near-extinction as a prelude to saving them.

A Botanical Christmas Card

If we really tuned in to plants, it is unlikely we would ever force valuable herbs to extinction. Granted, tuning in may seem difficult if we believe plants have nothing to communicate. But some plants seem to realize our difficulty in listening to them. They meet us halfway, and in certain situations make an extra effort to get their message across.

Sometimes the intimate connections between plants and people crop up when there is a profound need for them—as if the plant is standing by, ready to serve.

Consider what happened one harsh winter to academic philosopher Michael Grosso, which he describes in his provocative book *Soulmaking*.[40] One Christmas Eve, while Grosso was living in Edgewater, New Jersey, in a small brick house overlooking the Hudson River, the weather became bitterly cold and windy.[41] Although the mercury had dropped to zero and the roads were covered with a layer of ice, Francesca, Grosso's girlfriend, insisted on going to midnight Mass. So the two set out for the church, battling the frigid conditions.

Grosso found the ceremony disappointing—the crowd inattentive and disrespectful, the priest uninspiring. After returning home, Grosso and Francesca sipped hot tea in the cold house with their coats on. They exchanged gifts, but there was no joy in the ritual for either of them. Their relationship that night had turned as foul as the weather. Grosso slept on the sofa draped in his coat, too cold and numb to feel angry. "The spirit of Christmas was dead inside me," he recalls as he "dropped into a dreamless sleep."[42]

In the morning he was awakened by Francesca's sweet voice. Rousing himself on the sofa, he peered from under his coat to see her staring at the plant by the window. "Look! Look!" she said. "The plant flowered overnight!"

"What?" he mumbled, still sleepy.

"Your plant! Your plant bloomed!"

Grosso got up, walked to the window, and circled the plant. Francesa was right. Several white buds had appeared. He touched them and inhaled their fragrance with delight. Then his rational mind got the best of him and he began to stare at the blooming plant in disbelief. The small white buds seemed so out of place, out of time. Why should they have popped out when they were near freezing? Francesca took it all in stride. She stood over the plant, stroking the fat glossy leaves, sniffing the candy-sweet petals. "It's a Christmas card from heaven!" she said.

Grosso was baffled. It simply wasn't normal for a plant like that to bloom on the coldest day of the year, in the middle of the winter solstice, and on a Christmas morning. Disregarding his doubts, the buds developed into full flowers, gracing the entire apartment with a fragrance that was almost overwhelming. When the petals fell, he gathered them in a box.

He reminisced about the plant's history. He had bought the tropical plant a dozen years earlier while living in a loft in Chinatown. He tended it well and it grew big. One summer he left it in the care of students who forgot to water it, and the plant apparently died. But instead of discarding it Grosso nursed it back to life, and over the years it grew five feet tall. Although he moved often, he continued lavishing care on the plant, spritzing its leaves and tending the soil. When the plant bloomed on that frigid Christmas morning, it was as if it was saying "He was kind to me once. There now! I'll bloom and make him think of spring!"

Always the rationalist, however, Grosso continued seeking a naturalistic explanation for the plant's strange behavior. Further research revealed that *Dracaena fragrans* was a tropical shrub that flowered infrequently, normally requiring a tropical climate. He consulted two florists. One said he had never seen a *dracaena* flower, period—let alone in the cold, at night.

The other told Grosso a story that made him nervous. A customer once gave him her favorite cactus. She was elderly, frail, and too sick to care for it herself. About a year passed and the florist forgot about the woman. Then one day the cactus produced a beautiful red flower— the same morning the woman who gave it to him died.

Uneasy, Grosso repeated the story to a friend who was an opera lover, who countered with an equally strange happening. An opera star died one winter day. Snow had fallen during the night—and near his doorstep the next morning, the morning of his death, a red rose had bloomed. And beside the rose lay a dead songbird, fallen from the sky.

"These weren't the stories I wanted to hear," Grosso complained. So he sought out experts who might give him a naturalistic explanation. A biology professor could add little to what the florists had said, except he thought the whole affair was freaky. Finally, Grosso went to the world-famous New York Botanical Garden to consult with botanists and experienced horticulturists. All agreed that darkness and bitter cold were enemies of tropical plants. Besides, none of them had ever seen a *Dracaena fragrans* flower. One botanist declared it a "miracle."

"If there was no ordinary explanation, there was the possibility that we ourselves were the magical engineers who caused the plant to bloom," Grosso surmised. Perhaps, to compensate for his low spirits, he had somehow set the budding into motion, or perhaps he had done it with Francesca, unwittingly. "If this is the correct explanation, it implied a strange picture of what human beings may be capable of doing. It said something about unknown powers of the human soul, unknown instruments and avenues of influence." Or perhaps the plant *knew* that Francesco and Grosso were needy, and responded.

To which Grosso added one additional possibility. Perhaps there is something about "sacred time . . . holy days and healing times. Maybe the plant's bizarre behavior was caused by something above our individual, tribal, or species mind. By the mind, as some might say, of God. Maybe Francesca was right, and it really was a Christmas card from heaven."

Whither Green Medicine?

Everywhere people are asking how we can encourage the continued growth of "green medicine," the use of plants and herbs. The most counterproductive approach would be to regard green medicine in a purely pragmatic, utilitarian way, to consider herbs merely as the latest trick in our black bag: echinacea as the new penicillin, or ginkgo as the latest brain booster. Green medicine is not always "for" something.

It involves a respectful way of being in the world, in which the plant world is considered alive and sacred. It is about respect for all living things. So it is not specific therapies we wish to encourage, so much as green awareness. When the world is approached in this way, the plants come out to greet us, as we've seen. They announce themselves, and tell us how they can help.

The key question for us moderns, who are increasingly separated from the green world by the relentless asphaltification of the earth, is how to resuscitate the connections that were the living reality for our ancestors. It involves, as always, respectful invitation, humbly asking the green powers to manifest in our life, and placing ourselves in a position to hear plants when they speak. Unless we learn to do so, it is likely that the green world will recede from our medical culture once again, leaving us with the mechanistic medicine we are trying to transform.

One way of encouraging this process is to devise ways of letting green images grow within us. I've been having fun with this lately, trying to be a better listener to plants and trees. Following Kat Harrison's lead, I've been inviting green themes to show up in my dreams by putting a freshly plucked leaf under my pillow at night—tossing and turning over a new leaf, you might say. Thus far, my garden is not growing forty-pound cabbages like the gardens at Findhorn, Scotland, after they invoked the plant spirits to bless their barren patch of land. My garden, I suspect, has as many bugs as ever. But, increasingly, being green for me isn't about the size of the vegetables I grow or even about what I eat. And greenness isn't a color, but an attitude of the soul.

9

Bugs

I wish you all joy of the worm.

—*WILLIAM SHAKESPEARE, Antony and Cleopatra*

I magine a therapy that, when it is over, sprouts wings and flies away, leaving healing in its wake.

That's literally what happened in the case of a bedridden eighty-year-old patient of Dr. Grady Dugas of Marion, La. The elderly gentleman had severely infected pressure sores on his heels, hips, and buttocks, some an inch deep.[1] Antibiotics and debridement had proved ineffective, and Dr. Dugas figured he'd have to amputate both feet. Then the physician recalled that his diabetic grandmother had been treated successfully for infected ulcerations on her legs back in the 1930s with an unusual treatment— maggots, the worm-shaped larvae of flies. Thinking that he had nothing to lose, he contacted Jeffrey Wells, an entomologist at Lousiana State University. A week later Wells showed up in Marion with eight thousand blowfly eggs. Dugas applied the eggs to his patient's sores, just as he remembered in his grandmother's case. They hatched into larvae, ate the infected tissue, turned into flies, and flew off. Dugas applied more eggs and the process repeated itself. Four weeks later his patient's chronic bed sores were clean and were filling in with healthy tissue. Instead of amputating both the man's feet, Dugas sent him to a local hospital for skin grafts.

Lt. Kevin Shaeffer is also a believer in maggots. He was burned over 50 percent of his body when American Airlines Flight 77 hit his office at the Pentagon's Naval Command Center on September 11, 2001. Near death and on a ventilator, the burn surgeon successfully used maggots to clean up his damaged skin and reduce the chance of infection.[2]

That's what's possible when people feel kindly toward maggots. Often, however, these creatures strike terror in people's hearts—as on June 19, 2001, when eleven-year-old Vincent Ingram of Detroit, Michigan, bought a cheeseburger at a local McDonald's and took it home to eat.[3] Vincent alleges that when he chomped into the burger, it was infested with maggots. His attorney, who is representing Vincent in a $1 million lawsuit against McDonald's, describing the horror that gripped the Ingram household following Vincent's fateful meal, reported, "His sister is standing next to him and starts freaking out, because she sees these things crawling around . . . and out of his mouth."

Vincent's experience illustrates the instinctive revulsion most people have toward creepy-crawlies such as maggots, leeches, and worms. It wasn't always so. For example, "leech" is derived from the Gothic *lekesis*, meaning magician or healer, a clue to the reverence with which these creatures were once regarded.

Mythologies evolve, however, and today the awe our ancestors felt toward these creatures has largely disappeared. Currently we use their names as slurs or insults. When we call someone a leech, we are accusing him of being a parasitic, bloodsucking, selfish individual who attaches himself to another to get what he wants. To refer to someone as a worm is to consider him insignificant and unworthy of notice. To many people, worms and maggots are unspeakably low—invaders of corpses, emblems of destruction and death, mediators of rot and decay.

In view of the widespread disgust people feel toward maggots and leeches, one might presume that they had disappeared from the medical scene. But as Dalia Sofer, senior editor of the *American Journal of Nursing*,[4] says, "[T]he squeamish better toughen up. . . . *Hirudo medicinalis* [the medicinal leech] is back." It is not only to America's hospitals and clinics that leeches have returned. Sofer notes that they have "gone chic." Leech-containing cosmetics are now being sold in Europe, and a company in Dallas plans to market two million units of these creams annually in the United States. In addition to their use in cosmetics, plans are also being made to add leech components to toothpaste. These products take advantage of various pharmacological actions of *Hirudo medicinalis*, such as its anti-inflammatory, blood-thinning, vessel-dilating, and pain-relieving properties.

In fact, in August 2005, a federal board of medical advisors met to draw up regulations for how maggots and leeches should be safely grown, transported, and sold.[5]

Maggots: A Short History

The invasion of human wounds by worms is a condition called myiasis. The earliest recorded case may be the Old Testament story of Job, who lamented, ". . . my flesh is clothed with worms . . . my skin is broken, and become loathsome . . ."(Job 7:5, KJV)

The larvae of certain flies have long been used to treat suppurative wounds and clear away dead tissue. The ancient Maya of Central America soaked dressings in the blood of cattle and exposed them to the sun before applying them to wounds, expecting them to squirm in a few days with maggots. The Ngemba people of New South Wales, Australia, also used maggots to cleanse infected wounds, as did certain isolated tribes in the hills of Burma.[6]

The Western knowledge of the value of maggots is closely connected with warfare.[7] Ambroise Paré (1509–1590), chief surgeon to France's Charles IX and Henri III, reported firsthand in 1557 following the battle of St. Quentin that "the wounds of the hurt people were greatly stincking, and full of *wormes* with gangrene and putrifaction." He thought that the "wormes" were generated spontaneously from rotting flesh; he was unaware that they were connected with flies. Paré observed that one maggot-infested battlefield wound "recovered beyond all men's expectations," and is thus credited with the first European report recognizing the value of maggots in medical care.

Napoleon's great military surgeon, Baron Dominique-Jean Larrey, reported that during the Egyptian campaign most of the infected wounds became infested with maggots. The soldiers, he observed, were "much annoyed by the worms or larvae of the blue fly, peculiar to that climate." Larrey and his staff realized their value and tried to convince the soldiers that the maggots "cut short the process of nature" and speeded healing by removing necrotic tissue. Nevertheless, the French physicians made diligent efforts to rid the wounds of the larvae when changing bandages.[8]

Modern Developments

The first deliberate use of maggots in wound care is credited to John Forney Zacharias, a Confederate physician in the American Civil War. He wrote, "During my service . . . at Danville, Virginia, I first used maggots to remove the decayed tissue in hospital gangrene and with eminent satisfaction. In a single day they would clean a wound much better than any agents we had at our command. I used them afterwards at various places. I am sure I saved many lives by their use, escaped septicaemia, and had rapid recoveries."[9]

Credit for reviving interest in maggot therapy in the twentieth century is largely due to William S. Baer, a Baltimore surgeon who served in the army in World War I. Baer took care of two severely wounded men who had lain on the battlefield for seven days. Although their wounds were crawling with maggots by the time they reached the hospital, they were free of gangrene, infection, and fever. When Baer scraped away the maggots, he saw "the most beautiful pink granulation tissue that you can imagine." The experience deeply impressed him. Following the war, on his return to Johns Hopkins University School of Medicine as clinical professor of orthopedic surgery, he specialized in bone infections (osteomyelitis). In those pre-antibiotic days, chronic osteomyelitis was a vexing problem; it was not unusual for cases to drag on for a decade or longer in spite of aggressive surgical treatment, and mortality was high.

Hearkening back to the two battlefield cases that had riveted him, Baer decided on an experiment. He selected twenty-one individuals with chronic osteomyelitis, surgically removed all the dead tissue he could, stanched the bleeding, then filled them with as many maggots, produced by the local blowfly, as the wounds would hold. He replaced the maggots every four days for six or seven weeks. During this time the dead and dying tissue was consumed by the larvae and healthy pink replacement tissue took its place. Two months later, all twenty-one cases were totally healed. This was the most successful treatment of chronic bone infection then known to medical science.[10]

Government entomologists assisted these efforts by developing better methods of culturing the flies and ways of identifying the various look-alike species. It was crucial to use the correct one; one clinic had mistakenly bred screwworm flies, whose larvae destroy healthy, living tissue.

By the time Baer died in 1931, he had convinced a growing number of his colleagues of the value of maggot therapy. Between 1930 and 1940, around a hundred papers were written on the subject. Live maggots were being employed in more than 300 American and Canadian hospitals. Lederle Laboratories, the pharmaceutical giant, began the mass-production of sterile maggots and advertised their product in the *Journal of the American Medical Association.* The going rate was five dollars for one thousand (equivalent to about one hundred dollars today, but still inexpensive compared to the cost of most pills). Authorities were generally enthusiastic about the superiority of maggot therapy in a variety of conditions, mainly bone infections, abscesses, carbuncles, and leg ulcers.

In the 1930s, several researchers tried to isolate the "maggot active principle" from maggot extracts, the way they try to find the main ingredient in herbs today. An injectable maggot extract "vaccine" was tried, but was abandoned because of toxic reactions.[11]

Then, with the advent of sulfa drugs in the mid-1930s, penicillin in the 1940s, and advances in surgical techniques, maggot therapy became almost extinct. For more than forty years, the field fell silent.[12] Some took pride in laying maggots to rest. As one individual wrote, ". . . Fortunately maggot therapy is now relegated to a historical backwater, of interest more for its bizarre nature than its effect on the course of medical science . . . a therapy the demise of which no one is likely to mourn . . ."[13] The response was understandable. With antibiotics handy, who needed worms?

Maggot Renaissance

The reason for the resurgence of maggots is straightforward: the increasing resistance of microbes to antibiotics, the problem of failing immune systems in various illnesses, and a rising tide of chronic infections.

The most prominent champion of maggot therapy today is Ronald A. Sherman, assistant professor of medicine at UC-Irvine. As with Baer, serendipity played a role in Sherman's interest in maggot therapy. While working at the UCLA Medical Center in the 1980s, Sherman encountered a patient who came in with a leg wound crawling with worms. He and his colleague on the case, Dr. Edward Pechter, were initially disgusted. Then they noticed that healthy, uninfected tissue was growing into the wound. Although Pechter's enthusiasm waned, Sherman's grew; he has written definitive articles about maggot therapy and is the field's leading proponent.[14,15]

Sherman comes by his interest in maggots honestly. He was an avid bug collector as a child and holds a degree in entomology (the study of insects), as well as in medicine. He has been interested in the therapeutic uses of insects most of his life. Today he acts as a clearing house for information in this field and he handles queries from doctors from all over the world.

Sherman says that people don't think about maggot therapy until all other methods have continued to fail, which he finds irrational. Why delay maggot therapy? It's low-cost, requires no anesthesia, causes few to no side effects, and maggot-treated wounds heal with minimal scarring.

Getting started with maggot therapy is relatively simple. All you need is a hunk of meat and a few flies. Reporter Dawn Blalock, who visited Sherman and followed him around the hospital, wrote an article about his work for the *Wall Street Journal* describing what the maggot scene is like:[16]

> [H]e unlocks double doors . . . into his "insectary," essentially a maggot farm housed in a tiny converted kitchenette in the hospital's recesses. Thousands of blowflies buzz and swarm in three small cages holding putrid liver. The stench is overpowering— but maggots would rather starve than eat fresh food.
>
> The flies lay their eggs in the liver; left alone, the maggot eggs would hatch, engorge themselves and turn into flies. Dr. Sherman intervenes by removing the eggs from the liver and bathing them in a chemical solution that sterilizes them without killing them. After hatching, they are sewn into a patient's wound, which is sealed with a mixture of glue and gauze. This creates a little window allowing the maggots to breathe, and Dr. Sherman to observe them at work.
>
> Barely a millimeter long when they go into the wound, they come out two to three days later five to ten times bigger. Removing them is no problem: Feasting maggots become drowsy, reaching a state of near-hibernation.

Sherman has treated hundreds of patients since his first encounter with a maggot-infested wound. One was a Mr. Taylor, a 59-year-old carpet salesman who was hospitalized at the Veterans Affairs Medical

Center in Long Beach, California. Taylor was a diabetic with a gangrenous, ulcerated right leg due to compromised arterial blood flow. The gangrenous ulcer refused to heal and his surgeon was on the verge of amputating the leg. Following Sherman's intensive maggot therapy over several months, the gangrenous ulcer healed and Taylor kept his leg. [17]

The flies Sherman most often uses in maggot therapy are *Lucilia* species belonging to the family Calliphoridae, most commonly the "greenbottle" blowfly, *Lucilia sericata.* Their larvae are ideally suited to the task; if placed on healthy human tissue, they starve; if on necrotic tissue, they fatten and thrive. The larvae have to be "harvested" from wounds at the right time. If left to their own devices, they would turn into flies and fly away—not a welcome prospect in the hospital. They are disposed of following removal from the wound in the same way as other surgical dressings and infectious wastes.

Increasing Acceptance

Most doctors who use maggot therapy are pleased with the results— 95 percent in a British survey.[18] Acceptance by patients is also high.[19] This may be a surprise to healthy people who think worms are completely out of place in modern hospitals. But to patients facing amputation after conventional therapies have failed, any option can seem welcome. Said Taylor, the 59-year-old diabetic on the verge of losing his leg because of a gangrenous ulcer, "I tell you, my thoughts were, I don't want to lose my leg, let's take every shot." [20] And Edward Wicks, a 73-year-old former bombardier captain and car salesman, who resisted maggot therapy for a diabetic foot ulcer until his wife talked him into it, says, "They are creepy-crawly little rascals, but they sure do a job on infection. When the things were done with me, I was well." [21]

Whither Maggot Therapy?

In June 2003, the U.S. Food and Drug Administration (USFDA) approved the marketing of both maggots and leeches as medical devices. Although neither had been strictly prohibited, the FDA's imprimatur is likely to boost the clinical use of these organisms and stimulate research. But ironically, one of the problems for maggot therapy is that it is so inexpensive—*so* cheap, says Sherman, that the large pharmaceutical companies are unlikely to bankroll further research because they won't make much profit, even if clinical trials prove successful.[22]

Still, the future looks bright. As of 2000, around fifty centers in North America were using maggots in treating pressure sores, diabetic foot ulcers, infected surgical wounds, wounds infected with antibiotic-resistant ("flesh-eating") bacteria, burns, and traumatic injuries. In the U.K., the Biosurgical Research Unit in Bridgend, South Wales, has treated scores of patients and has distributed medicinal maggots for five thousand treatments to more than four hundred medical centers and general practitioners. Maggot therapy is also being used in institutions in Australia, Israel, Belgium, Germany, Sweden, Ukraine, and other countries.[23]

The World Health Organization suggests that by the year 2025, 228 million people in developing countries will suffer from diabetes,[24] resulting in countless cases of ulcers that can benefit from low-cost maggot therapy. Furthermore, new indications keep cropping up, such as the escalating numbers of injuries from land mines in war-ravaged, developing nations where conventional medical and surgical approaches are in short supply.[25] Tropical and rural regions in these countries are also likely to benefit from maggot therapy, because in these areas highly skilled surgeons and pharmaceutical options are often few and far between.[26]

One of the main challenges of maggot therapy in all parts of the world is how to improve its public image. Perhaps the best strategy is simply to continue doing good research and to publicize the findings not only in professional journals but in the popular media as well. And good studies are being done, such as a 2003 Swedish experiment in which seventy-four patients with chronic ulcers due to diabetes and other problems were treated with maggots with an 86 percent success rate and no serious side effects. The doctors found the therapy easy to use, and it was well accepted by the patients.[27]

Effective, convenient, low-cost, and acceptable to both patients and physicians: what more could one ask of any treatment?

The Return of the Leech

The public image of leeches, like that of maggots, has suffered mightily in modern times, particularly since Humphrey Bogart condemned them as "filthy little devils" in *The African Queen.*[28] But in spite of bad PR, leeches are making a comeback. They are being used to remove blood in situations in which swelling can interfere with healing, such as in skin grafting, breast reconstruction, or reattaching severed fingers. Substances found in the saliva of leeches are also proving useful, such as hirudin, which is used as a blood thinner.[29] In addition, an extract from the giant Amazon leech *Haementeria* is being tested as an inhibitor of metastatic lung cancer.[30]

The use of leeches for bloodletting dates back to the Stone Age. The rationale for bleeding a sick person was the belief that various maladies were caused by unwholesome blood, humors, and the like, and that health might be restored by ridding the body of impure blood.[31] Nicander of Colophon (200 BCE to 130 BCE) and Themison of Laodicea (123 BCE to 43 BCE) were among the first healers in recorded history to use leeches.

Knives, thorns, sharp stones, and even teeth faded in and out of popularity as methods of draining blood from the body. The British medical journal *Lancet* owes its name to a tool once used for bloodletting. Leeches eventually replaced sharp instruments such as lancets because they were believed to be less painful, and the amount of blood they removed was more controllable than when incisions were made.

We often imagine that bloodletting was a delicate affair that involved the release of small amounts of blood from the body, but often this was not the case. During the yellow fever epidemics that swept the United States in the late eighteenth century, a vigorous discussion occurred among doctors over the correct volume of blood that should be removed. Some advocated "bleeding to syncope"— passing out—and whether a patient should be bled until he fainted while lying down or standing up was a matter of intense debate.[32]

It is difficult to grasp how popular leeches once were in Europe and the United States. Between 1829 and 1836, five to six million leeches were used annually in the hospitals of Paris, draining its citizens of around 40,000 pounds of blood a year. At one time, 30 million of the most popular leech, *Hirudo medicinalis*, were imported from Hamburg to the United States, depleting Germany of this "irreplaceable medical apparatus."[33] The supply was so short that in 1835 a five-hundred-dollar offer was made to anyone who could breed European leeches in America. Enthusiastic leechers saw indications for bloodletting everywhere, including serious medical illnesses such as congestive heart failure, heart attack, meningitis, epilepsy, and embolism. One authority even advised applying leeches over an inflamed jugular vein as a treatment for polio.[34]

Leeches could be problematic. They had to be watched carefully to make sure they did not creep out of reach into body cavities where they could cause trouble.[35] If used in the vagina, they could migrate into the uterus; if on hemorrhoids, into the rectum; if in the head-and-neck area, they could attach to the pharynx and obstruct the airway when they swelled following engorgement with blood. Severe allergic reactions were always a concern.[36]

Practitioners were intrepid at getting leeches to do their bidding. A leech attached to the pharynx could be encouraged to loosen its hold and detach by gargling with salt water or vinegar. In using leeches to treat tonsillitis, the doctor often tied one end of a string to the leech and the other to his finger in order to maintain control of its position. When leeches were inadvertently swallowed, wine was a preferred remedy, although some authorities doubted a leech could survive a bath in gastric juices.[37] Oozing from the bite site was the most frequent complication. It could continue for twenty-four hours and could be difficult to stop. Compression or the use of cobwebs, burned rags, lint, silver nitrate, or the point of a red-hot knitting needle were used to stanch the flow. If these were unsuccessful, the bite could be excised and sutured. In people with bleeding disorders such as hemophilia, leeches could cause serious or fatal hemorrhage. If the same leeches were used to treat more than one patient, they could transmit infections such as syphilis. Infection could also result from the bite of an unsanitary leech.

Leeches could be finicky, and getting a leech to go to work was not always easy. It first had to be induced to attach itself to the patient. To tempt them, the skin was washed with warm or hot water to bring blood to the surface. Some authorities advised shaving the skin as well. If this didn't work, the skin was rubbed with a piece of raw meat or moistened with sugared water or milk. If the leech remained recalcitrant, the leecher could prick the skin of his patient or even his own finger and smear the blood over the area. To make sure the leech bit the right place, it could be applied via a cup that was inverted over the spot, or a hole could be cut in blotting paper that was then placed over the area of concern, exposing only the intended site. Applying the leech to an anatomically complex area such as a nostril or the throat could be difficult, and for this purpose a leech-glass—a tube open at both ends—was used.

Sometimes the leech got full after fifteen or twenty minutes and quit sucking before the desired amount of blood had been removed. To prompt it to go back to work, the Roman physician Galen advised puncturing or cutting off the tail of the leech so that it would lose blood itself and resume feeding; or the leech could be stripped by applying pressure from the tail forward, which forced the blood out of its mouth. If these methods failed, the leech could be submerged in a weak saline or vinegar solution, which caused it to regurgitate. How to get the leech to detach when it was still feeding? Table salt or vinegar did the job. Forceful removal was not advised; parts of the mouth could be left in place and a "phagodenic ulceration" could result.[38]

By the end of the nineteenth century, however, leeching was in decline. Medicine was changing rapidly, and science and technology

were in their ascendancy. Although popular for two millennia, belief
in the value of bloodletting as a shotgun approach to human illness
was fading, and leeching no longer possessed the cachet once associated with it. But it had been a glorious run.

As leeches crawled to the sidelines of the healing professions, the
practice of leeching seemed moribund. No one could have predicted
that the lowly leech would re-emerge a century later, smack in the
middle of the most high-tech medicine the world has ever seen.[39]

The most common use of leeches currently is to treat venous congestion, a stagnation of blood at surgical sites such as skin grafts. The
leech reduces swelling by swallowing blood, and an anticoagulant in
the leech's saliva prevents the sluggish blood in the surgical area from
clotting. Leeches essentially act as surrogate veins until the real blood
vessels heal and resume function. By improving circulation, leeches
make more oxygen available at the surgical site, speeding healing.

Leeches contain *Aeromonas* bacteria in their intestinal tract that
help digest the blood they swallow. Occasionally these bacteria
escape from the leech, enter a wound and cause infection. This problem prompted surgeon Nadine Connor and her colleagues at the
University of Wisconsin-Madison to design a mechanical leech. This
cup-sized device fits over a wound, continually bathes it with an anticoagulant solution, and provides gentle suction that keeps blood
seeping from the wound.[40]

Leeches also contain a local anesthetic in their saliva, which is why
their bites go unnoticed. German researchers have taken advantage of
this pain-dulling property by using leeches to treat painful arthritic
knees. Results indicate that a single leech treatment is more successful
in relieving pain during the ensuing week than daily applications of a
standard anti-inflammatory gel.[41]

Beyond the Yuck Factor

Maggots and leeches have fascinated me for a long time. A friend
of mine who is a psychoanalyst considers my curiosity about these

flesh-eating, bloodsucking creatures perverse. He finds all sorts of morbid, hidden meanings in my interest. He says that since worms will eventually have their way with us, my interest in maggots represents a death wish. I in turn accuse him of suffering from an overheated imagination. Can't a maggot just be a maggot?

To me there is something special about maggot and leech therapy, which one simply does not see with drugs and surgical procedures. When maggots and leeches go to work on us, all parties benefit: We get better and the creatures get a meal. There is a lovely symmetry here, a mutual advantage through cooperation, and we ought to pay more attention to such things.

We need to free ourselves from our revulsion toward maggots and leeches—what's been called the "yuck factor." Our turnoff is irrational. It makes no sense to reject a therapy that is inexpensive, almost completely free of side effects, and often highly effective when conventional treatments have failed.

Young children see the "bug world" differently from adults. They instinctively befriend frogs, toads, snails, turtles, worms, insects, and even snakes and spiders. They play with them, talk to them, give them names, take them home, construct lodging for them, and feed them. "For a year, my world as a little girl was a red coffee can, some sand, and a bunch of doodle bugs," reports literary agent Kitty Farmer. "That was before I moved on to fireflies and jelly jars." Kids will befriend and make pets out of almost any creature, often to their parents' dismay. A trip to a pet store to watch young children in wide-eyed attunement with other living things is well worth the visit. It all suggests an atavistic connection with the wild world, and that the "yuck factor" is not innate.

We *learn* to be offended by certain things. As environmentalist and educator Joanne Elizabeth Lauck observes in her book *The Voice of the Infinite: Revisioning the Insect-Human Connection,* "Disgust is, after all, a learned response. Every culture teaches its members what is disgusting and what is not. Children develop their disgust reaction by observing the facial expressions and reactions of their parents and teachers. And what is disgusting to members of one culture may not be disgusting to members of another. What allows us to eat shrimp and escargots, for example, and refuse maggots and caterpillars is the bias of our particular culture."[42]

The revulsion to maggots is not universal. Not only have maggots been used throughout history to promote wound healing, they have also been highly prized by indigenous peoples as food. The Dogrib Indians of the Athabaskan tribe of eastern Canada consider the maggots of several fly species a delicacy, as do many other native societies around the world. One reason is their nutritional value. Housefly maggots consist of 63 percent protein and 15 percent fat. They are so nutritious that entomologist Ronald Taylor advocates using maggots and insects to help alleviate world hunger. Because the majority of maggots feed on dead materials that are high in protein—animals, garbage, dung—Taylor suggests that mass-raised maggots could also help solve the world's burgeoning organic waste problem by converting these wastes into high-quality food supplements for domestic animals.[43,44]

A major reason for our phobia of maggots and leeches is our increasing separation from the natural world, the world of the wild. For increasing numbers of people, "nature" suggests a continual assault by invisible pathogens that require constant vigilance. This has led to "fortress medicine"—shielding ourselves from natural threats, many of which are imaginary, and developing aggressive ways of dealing with these challenges.

Maggot and leech therapy involves a different attitude toward nature—nature as ally, not as enemy—and a respect for the simple and the plain, the lowly and the commonplace.

This is an approach whose time has come. There is increasing evidence that a variety of primitive creatures can help us, and a new field in medicine—probiotics—is based on this premise. Probiotics, sometimes called "living drugs," are live micro-organisms that are used singly or in a mixture to improve an individual's microbial balance.[45] For example, certain strains of yeast have shown efficacy in clinical trials for preventing diarrhea following the use of antibiotics; *Lactobacillus* bacteria show promise as a treatment for urinary tract infections; and certain mouth bacteria inhibit strep throat and pneumonia. As we saw earlier in The Hygiene Hypothesis (pages 81–82), exposure to more germs in certain situations is valuable for immunity.[46]

A variety of bugs have been recruited in the fight against terrorism. Biologist Karen Kester, at Richmond's Virginia Commonwealth University, is spearheading the use of moths, crickets, bees, and maggots as biosentinels for detecting the release of toxic chemical and biological agents into the environment—a canary-in-the-mine approach. Kester's million-dollar project is funded by the Pentagon.[47]

Tarantulas are also in demand. Fred Sachs, professor of biophysics at the University of Buffalo's Center for Single Molecule Biophysics, and his research team have discovered a compound in the venom of the Chilean Rose tarantula that may prove useful in controlling conditions as diverse as cardiac arrhythmias, urinary incontinence, and muscular dystrophy. The Chilean Rose tarantula is about six inches wide and looks dangerous, but is harmless and is sold in the United States as a pet.[48]

A diet of microscopic worms or their eggs is proving to be one of the most effective treatments for inflammatory bowel disease (IBD), of which Crohn's disease and ulcerative colitis are the primary examples. In one clinical trial reported in 2004, a liquid concoction of pig whipworm eggs, drunk twice a month, resulted in a 50 and 70 percent remission rate for ulcerative colitis and Crohn's disease, respectively. This may prove to be a major breakthrough, because these diseases are currently incurable and can cause serious disability and death.

Why is the worm diet effective? As recently as the 1930s, 40 percent of American children had whipworms and roundworms in their gastrointestinal tract. As kids were increasingly de-wormed over the years, the incidence of IBD increased, prompting researchers to ask whether there might be a connection. Researcher Joel Weinstock, who is pioneering this therapy at the University of Iowa, theorizes that we've upset the balance between our immune system and parasites, which was worked out over millennia. "We're living in boxes, breathing sterile air and drinking sterile water," he says, and we are paying the price: our immune systems are now attacking not parasites, but our own digestive tract, resulting in IBD.[49,50]

Maggots and leeches unmask our unconscious attitudes toward the wild world, and they expose our prejudices about our role in the natural order. One such prejudice is our concept of the food chain, which we usually imagine as a vertical ladder with humans on top, eating anything below us that strikes our fancy. A more fitting symbol would be not a vertical chain but a circle, in which living things eat one another without any particular creature being on top. This process was captured by the American humorist and satirist Ambrose Bierce in his *The Devil's Dictionary*, with his circular definition of "edible":[51]

> *Edible, adj.* good to eat, and wholesome to digest, as a worm to a toad, a toad to a snake, a snake to a pig, a pig to a man, and a man to a worm.

When we employ maggots and leeches therapeutically, we invert the food chain and allow lower organisms to feed on us. Permitting primitive creatures to gnaw on us for a while—the diner becoming the dinner—requires a considerable dose of humility and takes some getting used to. Yet, as people continue to discover, a bruised ego is a fair price to pay when conventional treatments have failed.

10

Unhappiness

*No wonder Jung was later to tell me with a laugh that he
could not imagine a fate more awful, a fate worse than death,
than a life lived in perfect balance and harmony.*

—SIR LAURENS VAN DER POST

*People should be sufficiently discontented to feel
there is something to live for.*

—GEORGE BERNARD SHAW

I s happiness always good for us? Today, lots of therapies are
touted as having positive benefits on the body, mind, and spirit
—a sort of happily-ever-after effect. Are medical therapies supposed to make people happy? Is happiness always desirable?

George L. Engel, professor of medicine and psychiatry at the University of Rochester School of Medicine, has provided sobering evidence that happiness is not always compatible with health. Engel
collected 170 cases of sudden death over a six-year period and analyzed the psychological state of the individuals before their demise.
Although most of the fatalities were accompanied by negative emotions such as intense fear or depression, six percent were immediately
preceded by the experience of sudden happiness, such as receiving
good news.[1]

Happiness, clearly, can kill, and is not always a good thing. Is there a hidden calculus, according to which happiness and unhappiness are more complex than they seem?

"This Too Shall Pass"

Debra Denker, the international journalist, photographer, and documentary video producer who chronicled the Russian invasion of Afghanistan, encountered a charming tale during her sojourn with the Mujahedeen freedom fighters:

> There was once a king who commanded his wise men to make him a ring that would make him happy whenever he was sad, and sad whenever he was happy. They thought and thought, and finally decided that the ring should simply be engraved with the words, "This too shall pass."[2]

The lesson is unambiguous: happiness and unhappiness invariably succeed each other, as surely as night follows day. We cannot have it only one way.

Why is unhappiness so pervasive in our mental life? Why do we often become melancholy at moments when we least expect it, even when things are going well? Why do unhappy thoughts seem so easily to get the upper hand? These questions have been asked by every major religion, and answers have never been in short supply.

Our Predilection for Unhappiness

One might wonder whether we have some sort of biological predilection for negativity. In his admirable book, *The Evolving Self,*[3] Mihaly Csikszentmihalyi, professor and former chairman of the University of Chicago's Department of Psychology, offers several reasons why the mind seems to drift inevitably toward unhappiness. Consider those moments when our thoughts are unfocused and wandering randomly. At such times we might think there is an equal chance of settling on happy or unhappy topics, but this is not really so. Considering all the possible things about which we might think, the negative, depressing possibilities always seem to outnumber the positive ones. For example, if we think about our health, there is one positive scenario—good health— but hundreds of negative ones in the form of the various diseases that might befall us. If we think about moving into a new house, there is a single possibility that everything may be in working order, but innumerable chances that something might be out of whack—a leaky roof, faulty plumbing, a cracked foundation, infestation by termites, bad insulation, frayed wiring, and so on. If I think about an upcoming job interview, I might imagine that the interviewer will like me—a single possibility— but this may be swamped by the things he might not approve of: my clothes, hair style, vocabulary, or employment history. It is as if all our potential thoughts are a roulette wheel of possibilities, with only a single red, positive slot amid thousands of black, negative ones.[4]

Philosopher Alan Watts saw our natural penchant for unhappiness mirrored in great art and literature. Because we have a more highly developed ability to imagine the dark than the sublime side of life, Watts observed, the great Renaissance paintings of hell are almost always more captivating than those of heaven, which are generally boring in comparison. We may marvel momentarily at the sight of God touching man on the heavenly ceiling of the Sistine Chapel, but it is Rodin's *Gates of Hell* and the fiendish details of a Hieronymus Bosch painting that are spellbinding. So it is with many great literary works. Those that deal with human failings and tragedy fascinate us far more than descriptions of utopia.[5]

We profess to prefer the heavenly to the hellish, but this is hypocrisy. Consider the current debate about violence in the entertainment industry. As if we're not unhappy enough, we watch graphic images of tragedy continually being served up by the movie, television, and music industries. Politicians of every stripe, clawing for any advantage in the public mind, decry these images and urge the passage of legislation to protect our innocence. Is anyone fooled by this rhetoric? Although we object to the violence and mayhem, we stand in the movie lines without complaining, devour televised proceedings of double-murder trials, and can't wait until the latest blood-and-guts horror tale comes out in paperback. The truth is, we can't get enough of the negative messages.

Unhappiness and Survival

Philosopher Bertrand Russell was interested in the gloomy tendencies of humans. He wrote, "The late F. W. H. Myers used to tell how he asked a man at a dinner table what he thought would happen to him when he died. The man tried to ignore the question, but on being pressed, replied: 'Oh well, I suppose I shall inherit eternal bliss, but I wish you wouldn't talk about such unpleasant subjects.'"[6]

Why our predilection for morbid views? Csikszentmihalyi suggests that a pessimistic bias has been ingrained in our thinking through the long course of evolution. According to evolutionary theory, traits and behaviors that help an organism survive and reproduce tend to become built in biologically and perpetuated in subsequent generations. Unhappiness—not happiness, Csikszentmihalyi proposes—is more likely to help an organism survive in a hostile environment. If we dwell on negative possibilities, we will be more alert and poised to respond to dangerous events that could happen at any time. "By dwelling on unpleasant possibilities," Csikszentmihalyi states, "we will be better prepared for the unexpected." If this hypothesis is correct, the mind has become trained across our species' long history to turn toward negative thoughts, like a compass needle points northward.[7]

We see predilections for negative thought everywhere, as Csikszentmihalyi makes clear. Crowds gather at a street fight and congregate at a fire, rubberneckers tie up traffic on expressways when passing an auto accident, ambulance chasers risk their lives to get closer to tragedy. "Attention is attracted to violence and danger, whereas it skips over the normal, the peaceful, the contented."[8]

Thus do our newspapers and television relish tragedy and gore, always ready to oblige our tastes. "As a result," Csikszentmihalyi observes, "the average child is estimated to witness over seventy thousand murders on television before he or she grows up."[9]

The possible link between our biology and our fascination with the negative side of life raises interesting questions about religion. One of the characteristics of many Western religious views is their focus on the innate depravity of human beings and their need to be redeemed or somehow "saved." Could our collective religious fascination with the dark side of human nature be a holdover from our remote biological past? Do we find the image of intrinsic depravity more alluring than inner divinity because we have a built-in bias toward unhappiness? Are we destined by our DNA to be more enchanted by our weaknesses than our glory?

Not only do we focus naturally on the unhappy, negative side of life, sometimes negative events seem uncannily to seek us out. "A few years ago," Csikszentmihalyi relates,

> a Canadian professor . . . was planning retirement with his wife. Being sensitive and rational people, they decided to retire to the safest spot on earth they could find. They spent years poring over almanacs and encyclopedias to check out rates of homicide and health statistics, inquire about the directions of prevailing winds (so as not to be downwind of probable nuclear targets), and finally found a perfect haven. They bought a house on an island early in 1982. Two months later their house was destroyed: Their choice had been the Falkland Islands.[10]

These instances remind one of the adage, "Like attracts like"—a double whammy if ever there was one.

If our capacity to focus on negative possibilities and to be unhappy has given us a survival advantage in our evolutionary history, then unhappiness is a friend and ally deserving of our respect and gratitude. Were it not for our intrinsic capacity to feel sad, we might not be around to lament the fact that we are not always ecstatic. We might consider giving thanks the next time we feel down in the dumps, recalling that unhappiness has paved the way for happiness across the eons. This perspective might actually help us endure sadness, and might prevent us from becoming trapped in that pathetic, negative feedback loop of feeling unhappier about not feeling happy. If we realized the value of unhappiness in life—not just in our individual life but in the history of our species—we might be more balanced, more stable, and tougher. We might need less Valium.

Unhappiness and Modernity

In contrast, we have pathologized unhappy states of mind. The blather of Madison Avenue assures us that if we are not happy at every waking moment, there is something wrong. As physician-author Lewis Thomas, Sloan-Kettering's director of research for many years, put it,

> There's an awful lot of talk these days implying that it is abnormal to be unhappy . . . that if you're unhappy you ought to go see a doctor. . . . There's a whole new profession of people who advise other people on how to live a life. . . . This has been greatly overdone. There's a lot of genuine mental illness. . . . But it worries me that people, especially the young, are being brought up to believe that if they're unhappy, they ought to go see a counselor and get what's called guidance.[11]

The most common way of attempting to neutralize unhappiness is not through counseling, however, but through some form of instant gratification: a shopping spree, movies, alcohol, a party, or medication. Instead of trying desperately to annul our gloomy moments, could we learn to be with them, if ever so briefly? Could we honor the contribution negative states of mind have made to the evolution of our species and to our own existence? If we did so, we might find that the unhappy feelings would lighten of their own accord, as foretold by the inscription on the king's ring.

What have we lost in our rush to obliterate our melancholy moments? Are we losing the toughness needed to survive in a turbulent world by expecting always to be "blissed out" and serene? If the edge in the high-stakes game of survival belongs to the best-prepared and the most resilient—and if tolerance for unhappiness fosters these very abilities—we may be in for some rude surprises.

Today people speak of happiness as if it is a right. Our founding fathers took a different view. In the Declaration of Independence, they defended the pursuit of happiness, not happiness per se. They saw happiness as an ideal—something of great value, something to be realized if only we are wise enough—which is a much different attitude than the one that prevails today.

Unhappiness and Spirituality

Many spiritual traditions assure us that it is indeed "spiritually correct" to be unhappy from time to time. Unhappiness and happiness succeed each other like the seasons, and it is quite unnatural to be stuck permanently in some unchanging, tropical paradise of positive emotion. As a Zen saying puts it, "After ecstasy, the laundry." Some spiritual giants have actually seemed to turn away from the highest notes on the emotional scale. An example of that is St. Teresa of Avila, who, in a letter written in January 1577, said, "I've had raptures again. They're most embarrassing. Several times in public . . . during Matins, for instance. I'm so ashamed, I simply want to hide away somewhere!"[12]

A similar attitude is common in Buddhism. "[A] Zen master . . . after listening to one of his students report on the visions of Light and True Buddhahood that he had experienced during meditation, responded soberly, 'Keep meditating. It will go away.'"[13]

In a comparable story, one day it was announced by Master Joshu that the young monk Kyogen had reached an enlightened state. Much impressed by this news, several of his peers went to speak with him. "We have heard that you are enlightened. Is this true?" his fellow students inquired. "It is," Kyogen answered. "Tell us," said a friend, "how do you feel?"

"As miserable as ever," replied the enlightened Kyogen.[14]

Writer Natalie Goldberg relates an encounter with her Buddhist teacher, Katagiri Roshi, with whom she had previously studied for six years, which illustrates the appropriateness of negative emotions. When Goldberg finished her book *Writing Down the Bones* in Santa Fe in 1984, she felt the need to visit Roshi in Minneapolis again. She showed him the book and said, "Roshi, I need a teacher again. The people in Santa Fe are crazy. They drift from one thing to another."

"Don't be so greedy," he replied, shaking his head. "Writing is taking you very deep. Continue to write."

"But Roshi, it is so lonely."

"Is there anything wrong with loneliness?" he asked, lifting his eyebrows.

"No, I guess not."

The conversation went on to other things. Suddenly she interrupted him. "But Roshi, you have sentenced me to such loneliness. Writing is very lonely," she stressed again.

"Anything you do deeply is very lonely," he replied.

"Are you lonely?" she asked him.

"Of course," he answered. "But I do not let it toss me away. It is just loneliness."[15]

Frederick Douglass, one of America's towering black leaders of the nineteenth century, spoke about the polarities inherent in life:

> If there is no struggle, there is no progress. Those who profess to favor freedom, and yet deprecate agitation, are men who want crops without plowing up the ground. They want rain without thunder and lightning. They want the ocean without the awful roar of its many waters. This struggle may be a moral one, or it may be a physical one, or it may be both moral and physical— but it must be a struggle.[16]

Many great wisdom traditions have regarded unhappiness and suffering as steps toward wisdom. Mythologist Joseph Campbell affirmed this view, stating that human beings become wise in two ways. They may experience a sudden, unbidden revelation—an epiphany or "instant enlightenment"—or they may suffer, which is far more common. To limit unhappiness, therefore, is to block one of the major pathways toward wisdom. And if the suffering is fully entered and engaged, it can be transformed, as many wise spiritual teachers maintain.

An example comes from the life of Sri Ramana Maharshi, perhaps the most beloved saint of modern India. Maharshi was afflicted with cancer at the end of his life, and he would cry out in pain at night. His screams often prevented those who had come to study at his ashram from sleeping. Some of his devotees, wanting to put the best possible face on things, insisted that their teacher was not really in pain but was using "yogic control." On hearing this rationale, Maharshi objected. "There is pain," he explained, "but there is no suffering"—a reminder that pain and serenity can coexist and are not required to annihilate each other.

A Challenge to Healers

If unhappiness plays a positive role in life, it does not mean that more is always better. Excessive melancholy can shade into depression, which can overwhelm and destroy. But just as we can have too much unhappiness, we can also have too little. Life needs to push back; we need resistance if we are to build strength and stamina on the mental as well as the physical plane.

It is easy to criticize the tendency in modern culture to rid ourselves of unpleasantness through the mindless consumption of material luxuries and, when this doesn't work, to complete the job by altering our consciousness with alcohol, drugs, and other chemicals. It is also easy to castigate modern medicine for doing the same through the wholesale prescription of tranquilizing medications.

Moreover, therapists who use alternative or complementary forms of treatment often fall into the same trap. "Natural" therapies can be used as vigorously as pharmaceuticals to eradicate pain and unpleasantness. Alternative therapists, no less than orthodox clinicians, need to make a place in their conceptual models for suffering and unhappiness. All of us physicians, whether conventional or alternative, must resist the reflex tendency to obliterate every ounce of discomfort for those we serve. We ought to help our patient-clients explore the role of unpleasantness in their lives, and we must be patient while this process proceeds at its own pace. Above all, we should resist equating healing with feeling good. This is a difficult lesson for healers; we prefer that our patients always be happy. But unless we understand the place of unhappiness in the lives of those we serve, we shall have to endure more unhappiness ourselves, for that is the price always paid for severing the wholeness that is healing.

11

Nothing

It was nothing, but *nothing* isn't an absence,
it's a presence.

—BARBARA KINGSOLVER, *Prodigal Summer*

Growing up, when my twin brother and I misbehaved, which was most of the time, and Mom demanded, "What are you boys doing?" we invariably replied, "Nothing." Our little lie usually worked. I therefore learned early on that nothing had, as biologists say, survival value or at least could prevent punishment, which to my brother and me were pretty much the same thing. This meant that nothing was actually something—my first exposure to paradox.

Webster's defines nothing as that which is nonexistent, insignificant, unimportant, trivial, useless, or empty, all of which reflect our culture's blindness to the value and power of nothing. In America, to achieve nothing is to fail. If we stand for nothing or believe in nothing, we are considered cowardly and weak-willed. We equate doing nothing with sin itself: "Idle hands are the devil's workshop." When nothing makes a token appearance—as in the lyric from *Porgy and Bess*, "I got plenty o' nuttin', and nuttin's plenty fo' me"—no one takes it seriously. When someone actually celebrates nothing and not-doing as a way of life, such as bohemians, beats, and hippies, they are generally considered subversive and are marginalized by the wider culture.

Not-Doing

Not-doing has fallen on hard times, particularly in modern medicine.[1] Yet when Hippocrates, the father of Western medicine, said that the first goal of a physician was to do no harm, he was implying that doing nothing might sometimes be the wisest course of action. We physicians have largely abandoned Hippocrates' endorsement of a minimalist approach to healing. We tend to consider nature as failure-prone, one big accident waiting to happen. Disease is always lurking and pathology is just around the corner. As a third-year medical student once put it, "A healthy person is someone who has not been completely worked up." Or as another pessimistic wag said, "Life is a sexually transmitted disease with 100 percent mortality."

Believing we can invariably improve on nature, we physicians have become incorrigible doers and meddlers. Every day we intrude into our patients' lives without any clear-cut justification for doing so, often causing unspeakable harm. Doing nothing remains one of the most difficult things we physicians ever attempt. Sometimes I think board certification in not-doing should be a legal requirement for the practice of medicine.

Arguments over the extent to which physicians ought to intervene in people's health are nothing new. As physician Andrew Weil, director of the Program in Integrative Medicine at the University of Arizona in Tucson, observes in his book *Spontaneous Healing*,[2] "Doctors believe that health requires outside intervention of one sort or another, while proponents of natural hygiene maintain that health results from living in harmony with natural law. In ancient Greece, doctors worked under the patronage of Asklepios, the god of medicine, but healers served Asklepios's daughter, the radiant Hygeia, goddess of health."

Spontaneous Remission

The most dramatic example of the ability of the body to heal when little or nothing is done is when dreaded diseases such as cancer simply go away.

The most comprehensive look at this "epidemiology of nothing" is the landmark *Spontaneous Remission: An Annotated Bibliography*[3] by Brendan O'Regan and Caryle Hirshberg of the Institute of Noetic Sciences in Petaluma, Calif. These authors summarize 1,385 published case reports or series of cases in which cancer and other serious illnesses disappeared without any treatment, or with treatment believed insufficient to produce a cure. Often these remissions followed periods in which the patients and physicians did precisely nothing, engaging in what doctors call "benign neglect."

An example published in 1990[4] involved a sixty-three-year-old Caucasian woman who was admitted to the hospital with a four-month history of abdominal discomfort and nausea, a seven-pound weight loss, and a mass in her right upper abdomen. Her liver function blood tests were deranged and her chest X ray showed scattered lesions believed to be cancer metastases. An ultrasound study showed lesions suggestive of tumor throughout her liver. A liver biopsy resulted in a diagnosis of a primary hepatocellular carcinoma, a type of cancer that has a very poor prognosis with a mean survival time of around six months. She was discharged home to die without therapy, because no treatment was considered worthwhile.

Five months later all her symptoms had disappeared and she had gained nearly seven pounds. Her chest X ray showed disappearance of the metastases and her liver function tests were normal. A repeat ultrasound study of her liver showed considerable shrinkage of the original abnormal areas, and a liver biopsy showed only scar tissue without any evidence of cancer. A year following her diagnosis she remained well, continued to gain weight, had no symptoms, and her liver function tests remained normal.

O'Regan and Hirshberg call these events "an epidemiological

unknown."[5] You'd think these cases would be studied in depth instead of being ignored, but they are not. Physicians often have an aversion to such events; I know of patients who were turned away by their doctor after they underwent a remission following doing nothing. Ignoring these cases is astonishing, and illustrates the horror with which we physicians have come to regard not-doing.

Fortunately, not all doctors hold these events in disdain. One prominent physician who saw the value of do-nothing spontaneous remissions was Lewis Thomas. As he put it,

> The rare but spectacular phenomenon of spontaneous remission of cancer persists in the annals of medicine, totally inexplicable but real, a hypothetical straw to clutch in the search for cure. . . . It is a fascinating mystery, but at the same time a solid basis for hope in the future: If several hundred patients have succeeded in doing this sort of thing, eliminating vast numbers of malignant cells on their own, the possibility that medicine can learn to accomplish the same thing at will is surely within the reach of imagining.[6]

But doing nothing is relative. What appears to be nothing to a physician may not be nothing to a patient. What, for example, did the sixty-three-year-old woman in the above case experience when she was sent home without therapy to die? What was going through her mind? It is impossible to know from reading the actual case report in the journal *Gut*, whose name is a clue to its physical orientation. Medical journals are a virtual blackout about what doing nothing means from the patient's point of view. If interventions are not physical, they usually aren't reported in scholarly write-ups.

In their book *Remarkable Recovery*,[7] Caryle Hirshberg and Marc Ian Barasch investigated what doing nothing meant to around four dozen patients who recovered from cancers that should have been fatal. They asked them their personal opinions about why they recovered. They found that the leading factor to which patients attributed their cure was prayer (68% of cases). Other factors were meditation (64%), exercise (64%), guided imagery (59%), walking (52%), music/singing (50%), and stress reduction (50%). When they inquired what psychological factors the patients felt were important in their recovery, the ones most often mentioned were belief in a positive outcome (75%), a fighting spirit (71%), acceptance of disease (71%), and seeing disease as a challenge (71%). Seventy-five percent reported benefit from artistic pursuits at which they were somewhat proficient, and 68 percent described experiencing feelings they could not rationally explain but which seemed important.

The value of not-doing surfaces in surprising contexts, such as in the management of childhood obesity, which is epidemic in the United States. Recent findings suggest that mothers who worry about their children's weight and intervene in their eating habits may actually make matters worse.[8] Imposing rules and strategies for eating interferes with the natural ability of kids to self-regulate their food intake, resulting in fatter children. But when a mother backs off and permits her child to eat everything on his or her plate, the child's total body fat is generally reduced.

Active intervention also backfired in a controlled study involving nine Veterans Affairs Medical Centers,[9] in which researchers assigned 1,396 hospitalized patients to one of two groups—one that would receive usual care for six months following discharge, or one that would receive intensive attention plus primary care for the same duration. The increased attention resembled the kind of care available in most HMOs—ready access to a nurse, a family doctor in charge of their case, and reminders of appointments and follow-up phone calls. The researchers predicted that intensive primary care would keep the patients healthier, reduce hospital readmissions by at least a third, and save money. But after six months hospitalizations actually rose by a third and there were 25 percent more deaths in the group getting the extra attention. "We were more surprised than anybody," said Morris Weinberger, MD, of the VA Hospital in Indianapolis, one of the directors of the study. "Instead of conferring benefit, closer scrutiny of the patients simply led to more medical care and perhaps to harm," said H. Gilbert Welch, MD, of Dartmouth Medical School.[10] "We can no longer assume that early intervention is always the right thing to do."

As in health care, so in daily life: common-sense ideas based in doing often produce unintended consequences. Consider the fact that people in increasing numbers are fleeing urban areas to the suburbs to escape crime. Risk analysts have determined that the chance of dying in a car accident in the United States exceeds the risk of dying from violent crime. Thus the urban escapees incur more risk due to increased driving time than if they'd stayed put. In the attempt to outrun one problem, they run headlong into another.[11]

Emptiness

Some cultures have actually championed the value of nothing, none more so than the ancient Taoists. Lao Tsu, a contemporary of Confucius in the sixth century BCE, laid the foundation for Taoism in the *Tao Te Ching*, a collection of his teachings. The Taoist approach emphasizes the implicit wisdom of nature, called Tao or the Way, and is profoundly respectful of nothingness and not-doing. An example:

> *Thirty spokes share the wheel's hub;*
> *It is the center hole that makes it useful.*
> *Shape clay into a vessel;*
> *It is the space within that makes it useful.*
> *Cut doors and windows for a room;*
> *It is the holes which make it useful.*
> *Therefore profit comes from what is there;*
> *Usefulness from what is not there.*[12]

And,

> *In the pursuit of learning, every day something is acquired.*
> *In the pursuit of Tao, every day something is dropped.*

Less and less is done
Until non-action is achieved.
When nothing is done, nothing is left undone.[13]

A Westerner who saw the value of not-doing and non-interference was psychologist C. G. Jung. Some problems, Jung believed, have a way of solving themselves. He said,

> I have often seen individuals who simply outgrew a problem which had destroyed others. . . . Some higher or wider interest arose on the person's horizon, and through the widening of his view, the insoluble problem lost its urgency. . . . What, on a lower level, had led to the wildest conflicts and emotions full of panic, viewed from the higher level of the personality, now seemed like a storm in the valley seen from a high mountain-top. This does not mean that the thunderstorm is robbed of its reality; it means that instead of being in it, one is now above it.[14]

In contrast, we believe we must *do* something if we're unhappy. An industry consisting of self-help programs and support groups for every conceivable problem has arisen, whose sole purpose is to tell us what to do to feel better and function more productively. If all else fails, we can medicate our mental sufferings out of existence with a blizzard of tranquilizers and antidepressants designed to steel us against the barbs of life. The message implicit in all these approaches is that problems always go from bad to worse. Spontaneous decay, not spontaneous healing, has become our credo.

The Dark Side of the Bean

It is remarkable how many of the rituals of our daily life are a flight from nothing and not-doing. Take our passion for coffee and caffeine, the most widely consumed drug in America. Writer Amanda Huron[15] describes how coffee did not become an American tradition until office work became the norm. Coffee was advertised to employers as a way to make their employees happier and more productive, and the "coffee break" took hold.

Huron is one of the millions of Americans who have zero tolerance for not-doing. "I've always hated that sluggish feeling that creeps up on me sometimes—that feeling of not really wanting to do anything, of just wanting to lie around and shut my mind off," she says. She began using coffee as an antidote to the empty spaces and down times that are a part of everyone's daily life. It worked: "It used to be that when I felt that way, I'd just drink some coffee and presto, insta-energy."

Her insight into what she calls "the dark side of the bean" came when she started working at a coffee shop. Bleary-eyed customers would line up every morning beginning at 6:30 AM on their way to work. Huron realized she was a drug pusher. Her job was "to dole out drugs. . . . They [could not] make it through the day without me. . . . I [gave] them the strength and inspiration they [needed]. I [fed] them caffeine."

Huron began to question her own love affair with coffee. Her appetite for it gradually diminished and she evolved an ethos of not-doing:

> [N]ow I'm rethinking my attitude toward those low-energy, bored times. Maybe feeling bored and lazy isn't necessarily a bad thing. . . . In reality, we should sleep more and pack less into our days—or else change our lives so that we spend time doing things that are truly meaningful to us. I'll make no pretense of giving up coffee for good. . . . But I also want to know that I can get stuff done without it. And I want to value being a slug sometimes . . .

Colossal-Speak

Our vocabulary also reveals our aversion to nothing, the minimal, the plain.

Consider, for instance, how we use inflated adjectives. "The trend in everyday conversation," says writer Ray Nedzel, "is to use grandiose words.[16] 'Outstanding!' is the new 'good,' 'amazing!' is the new 'OK,' and 'huge!' is the new 'big.'" Nedzel describes a recent experience in a Washington, D.C., restaurant. When he asked, "How's the salmon?" the waiter responded, "Fantastic!" Did it come with rice? "Absolutely!" Superlatives had overcome the server, when a "good" and a "yes" would have been sufficient.

This sort of escalation is epidemic. At Starbucks, Nedzel notes, the smallest coffee you can buy is a Tall. A medium-size coffee is a Grande, which means large in Italian and Spanish. Neither can you purchase a small or medium drink at your local 7-Eleven, where your only choices are a Big Gulp, Super Big Gulp and Extremely Big Gulp. Nedzel has discovered that many of the chain clothing stores have also redefined sizes upward. What used to be a small is now a medium, a medium has become a large, and so on up the ladder. The trend is irritating; it makes you think you've gained weight, even if you haven't.

Why has everything become "awesome"? Nedzel says,

> [T]he reason for all this colossal-speak is clear: We are bored with our fantastic, wonderful lives. We want the next-next thing now. Now!... Everything can't be great... If everything is outstanding, if everything is the most amazing thing ever, is anything ever amazing at all?...
>
> Have people forgotten what it's like to be OK? Simply OK with what they have and who they are?

One way to defang colossal-speak, says Nedzel, is simply to pay attention and tell the truth. The next time someone asks, How are you, notice whether you respond with "Great!," "Terrific!," or "Fantastic!," and whether or not a simple "Fine" or "Okay" would be a more honest answer. If we can gear down a notch or two, we'll have words in reserve when we need to describe life's genuinely delicious moments.

And as we wean ourselves off the need to inflate everything by the words we use, we might find ourselves becoming more sensitive to life's minimalist moments, more appreciative of the nothing side of life.

Varieties of Nothing

Most of us harbor a deep need for simplicity. When our life becomes too busy and confused, an inner compass kicks in and reminds us that we need to rein in our behaviors and appetites to some minimal standard. Over the years each of us develops a repertoire of small anchors—varieties of nothing—that help us stay sane in a mad world.

Consider fashion. A subtle way of staying in touch with nothing involves the colors we choose for our clothes. As author Simon Garfield notes in his award-winning book *Mauve*, which charts the discovery of aniline dyes in the mid-1800s and their profound influence on Western civilization, current fashion designers know that in the United States "seventy to ninety percent of all sales are always black, all the year round. Followed by grey and navy." The goal of the fashion industry is to dictate the color makeup of the remaining ten percent.[17]

Black objects absorb all the wavelengths of the spectrum, reflecting nothing to stimulate a visual sense of color. Thus one of the dictionary meanings of black is "complete darkness or absence of light."[18] In a culture gone color-crazy, why the overwhelming preference for black, the nothing color, for personal adornment? The reason, I suggest, is that this is an area in which it remains socially acceptable to express our need for nothing—for understatement, simplicity, the freedom from affectation.

Doing nothing manifests also in creativity. Walt Whitman was a supreme example. He was an incorrigible do-nothing and a wanderer—he called it "loafing"—who transformed Western poetry. *Newsweek* columnist Anna Quindlen would have understood Walt's rambling tendencies. In her essay "Doing Nothing Is Something," she writes, "I don't believe you can write poetry, or compose music, or become an actor without downtime, and plenty of it, a hiatus that passes for boredom but is really the quiet moving of the wheels inside that fuel creativity."[19] Quindlen is concerned about American kids, who no longer know how to loaf. Their lives have become burdened with what she calls "the sheer labor of being a perpetually busy child." Children have become so busy, Quindlen reports, that many parents, oddly enough, are resorting to scheduling unscheduled time into their schedules, time that is dedicated to doing nothing in particular. An example is Ridgewood, New Jersey, where Family Night has been instituted, one night a week where there is no homework, athletic practices, or after-school events. And in Omaha, Nebraska, a group of parents has lobbied for increased recess.

How did this situation come to pass? Adults brought it about, says Quindlen, out of concern that if their children were not perpetually occupied in soccer leagues, acting classes, or with tutors, they would not be prepared to compete down the line with other busy kids for good colleges and jobs. "Let me make a suggestion," says Quindlen, "for the kids involved: how about [doing] nothing? There is . . . ample psychological research suggesting that what we might call 'doing nothing' is when human beings actually do their best thinking, and when creativity comes to call. Perhaps we are creating an entire generation of people whose ability to think outside the box . . . is being systematically stunted by scheduling."

Spirituality: Nobody Doing Nothing

When we genuinely acquire the knack of nothingness, we become in a sense a nobody. Many spiritual traditions tell us that transcending the ego and becoming a nobody reveal the greatest discovery of all: indwelling divinity. As the Hindu aphorism says, *"Tat tvam asi"*— "Thou art that."

In the annals of healing, no one glimpsed the idea of "the god within" more clearly than Florence Nightingale (1820–1910), the founder of modern secular nursing.[20] In 1872, she wrote:

For what is mysticism? Is it not the attempt to draw near to God, not by rites or ceremonies, but by inward disposition? Is it not merely a hard word for "The Kingdom of Heaven is within"? Heaven is neither a place nor a time. There might be a Heaven not only here but now. . . . Where shall I find God? In myself. That is the true Mystical Doctrine.[21]

In his classic volume *The Perennial Philosophy*,[22] philosopher and novelist Aldous Huxley affirmed the need for self-transcendence in realizing one's inner divinity. "[This] knowledge," he said, ". . . can come only to those who are prepared to 'die to self' . . ."

But the quest of awakening to our intrinsic divinity contains a paradox. If the divine is already within us, there is nothing to do to attain it. Thus the emphasis in many traditions on not-doing—stripping away all religious overlay and doctrinal beliefs in order to perceive what has been present all along. Self-transcendence and cessation of activity—nobody doing nothing—are the keys to this understanding. No wonder that in Buddhism the great sages were said to erupt in laughter upon this realization.

Throughout history, becoming a nobody has often been likened to becoming a fool. "Fool" is derived from the Latin *follis*, meaning a windbag, a container holding nothing. Having transcended the self, the fool has penetrated to the divine essence. Lacking an ego, he or she has nothing to lose by appearing stupid and inept.

Mark Twain, America's great fool, seemed to understand these connections. In an 1877 letter to William Dean Howells, he wrote, "I am a great & sublime fool. But then I am God's fool, & all His works must be contemplated with respect." [23]

Silence

One of the most endangered varieties of nothing in the modern world is silence. In a scathing observation, Huxley noted:

The twentieth century is . . . the Age of Noise. Physical noise, mental noise and the noise of desire—This din goes deeper, of course, than the ear-drums. It penetrates the mind . . .—news items, mutually irrelevant bits of information, blasts of corybantic or sentimental music, continually repeated doses of drama that bring no catharsis, but merely create a craving for daily or even hourly emotional enemas.[24]

Mark Twain agreed. "Noise proves nothing," he observed. "Often a hen who has merely laid an egg cackles as if she had laid an asteroid."[25]

Silence—whether called quietude, contemplation, meditation, or some other term—has been universally valued as an antidote to our noisy, chattering mind, so that deeper truths can be revealed. As author Carlos Castaneda writes, "Whenever the dialogue stops, the world collapses and extraordinary facets of ourselves surface, as though they have been kept heavily guarded by our words."[26] The spiritual writer Satprem advocates extending silence to thought itself: "[I]f the power to think is a remarkable gift, the power not to think is even more so."[27] We find the same message in the writings of Lao Tsu: "He who knows does not speak/He who speaks does not know."[28] St. John of the Cross agrees: "For whereas speaking distracts, silence and work collect the thoughts and strengthen the spirit."[29]

These comments, spanning nearly three millennia, reveal the great value all mystical traditions attribute to silence.

Silence of mouth and mind is one of nothing's greatest paradoxes. By thinking and saying nothing, we apprehend everything. Thus, historian of religions Edward Carpenter notes,

Of all the hard facts of science, I know of none more solid and fundamental than the fact that if you inhibit thought and persevere, you come at length to a region of consciousness below or behind thought, and different from ordinary thought in its nature and character. . . . [It is a world in which] one's soul is in touch with the souls of all creatures. It is to be assured of an indestructible and immortal life and of a joy immense and inexpressible.[30]

Again the message is the same: If this "joy immense and inexpressible" is to be realized, we must become nothing and nobody—a state in which, as Huxley says,

> ... there is no separate selfhood to obscure or refract ... the "white radiance of Eternity." ... The Thing in itself *can* be perceived—but only by one who, in himself, is no-thing.[31]

In contrast, our entire culture is dedicated to the task of turning nobodies into somebodies. Take the advertising industry, for example. Its goal is to inflame our desire to stand out, to be unique and different and over the top, because, frankly, we're wonderful and nothing is too good for us or beyond our reach. As the ads for military service put it, "Be all that you can be." And there are hundreds of ads based on flattery, such as "You deserve a break today"—the McYou message that appeals to that special you-know-who, who merits a you-know-what, at you-know-where.

From the perspective of the spiritual traditions mentioned above, fluffing up the ego guarantees not self-development but developmental arrest. But if we can transcend the ego and become nobody, magic happens. A new dimension of experience becomes possible, described by poet William Blake in his *Auguries of Innocence*:

> To see a world in a grain of sand,
> And a heaven in a wild flower,
> Hold infinity in the palm of your hand
> And eternity in an hour.[32]

There is a final seduction that awaits anyone who sees the world as it really is—the pride of enlightenment, of having finally achieved nobodyness. But, of course, pridefulness wrenches one back into being a somebody all over again. Therefore many spiritual traditions go to great lengths to emphasize that *everything* must be given up, and that nothing really does mean nothing. Thus Jesus' words in John 12:24: "Verily,

verily I say unto you, Except a corn of wheat fall into the ground and die, it abideth alone: but if it die, it bringeth forth much fruit." This process even requires dying to the beliefs and values the ego previously found helpful. As scholar of religions Ananda Coomaraswamy puts it:

> However far one may have gone [on the spiritual path], there remains a last step to be taken, involving a dissolution of all former values. . . . There always remains a last step, in which the ritual is abandoned and the relative truths of theology denied.[33]

Sri Ramana Maharshi said, "There will come a time when one will have to forget all that one has learned."[34] And a Zen aphorism urges, "Fish with a straight hook!"—the hook that catches nothing.

Pure Consciousness

Modern medicine does not look kindly on blank minds. Psychiatrists regard someone who has "lost their mind" as insane, and neurologists equate a state of mental nothingness with being unconscious or brain-dead. But in some spiritual traditions a state of complete mental emptiness is regarded as "pure consciousness," and achieving such a condition is considered a supreme achievement. W. T. Stace, the scholar of mystical traditions, describes this condition:

> Suppose that having got rid of all sensations, one should go on to exclude from consciousness all sensuous images, and then all abstract thoughts, reasoning processes, volitions, and other particular mental contents; what would there then be left of consciousness? . . . The introvertive mystics—thousands of them all over the world—unanimously assert that they have attained to this complete vacuum of particular mental contents, . . . a state of *pure* consciousness—"pure" in the sense that it is not the consciousness of any empirical content. It has no content except itself.[35]

Author Peter Russell, who earned degrees in theoretical physics, psychology, and computer science from the University of Cambridge, has explored this dimension of consciousness for three decades. He states:

> Indian teachings call this state *samadhi*, meaning "still mind." In samadhi there is awareness—one is awake—but there is no object of awareness. . . . [I]n samadhi there is the light of pure consciousness, but nothing else. It is the faculty of consciousness without any content.[36]

Although these mental states are associated with eastern spiritual traditions such as Buddhism, Hinduism, and Taoism, they are universal. As Russell says, "Similar descriptions can be found in almost every culture of the world."[37]

This point deserves emphasis. Today an increasing number of individuals hunger for spiritual experiences that have a mystical flavor, and many believe the only place they can find them is in the traditions of the Orient. Yet one of the finest explorations of mysticism ever written deals with the western Christian mystical tradition—Evelyn Underhill's classic volume *Mysticism*.[38] First published in 1911 and still in print, this great work remains current. Unfortunately, many Westerners are completely unaware that a vibrant mystical tradition exists within Christianity. Underhill shows otherwise. She explores the great Christian mystics and compares their insights with representatives from esoteric traditions worldwide. The views of the mystics are consistent across cultures, which is why it is said that all mystics come from the same country and speak the same language.

In his landmark work *The Religions of Man*, philosopher Huston Smith relates the experience of a Zen meditator whose awareness of self expanded to a sense of unity with all there is:

> Ztt! I entered. I lost the boundary of my physical body. I had my skin, of course, but I felt I was standing in the center of the cosmos. . . . I saw people coming toward me, but all were the same

man. All were myself. I had never known this world before. I had believed that I was created, but now I must change my opinion: I was never created; I was the cosmos; no individual . . . existed.[39]

What does this actually feel like? Smith says, "The mystical experience, . . . wherever it appears, in Zen or any other religion, brings joy, a feeling of oneness with all things and a heightened sense of reality which cannot be adequately translated into the language of the everyday world."[40]

Critics often dismiss these experiences as "dreamy mysticism" and warn that they will lead to a withdrawal from the practical side of life. But the opposite is generally true. The experience of pure consciousness fills the individual with compassion and love, which are a springboard for a fuller, more active participation in the world. Thus the Western tradition of the "practical mystic," represented by individuals such as St. Francis, Mother Teresa, and Florence Nightingale, who dedicated their lives to serving those in need.[41]

Buddhist scholar and physicist Alan Wallace, drawing on the language of physics, calls the state of mental emptiness "vacuum consciousness." He states, "Buddhist contemplatives have used vacuum states to investigate the nature of the mind for 2,500 years, a lot of lab time."[42] You'd think that this cumulative experience would carry weight with modern investigators of consciousness, but some breezily dismiss it. For instance, philosopher Barry Dainton of the University of Liverpool says,

If pure consciousness in this form *is* possible—if thousands or millions of people have known consciousness in this form— should we conclude that a bare Awareness is not only possible but actual? I think not. . . . I very much doubt whether these modes can be equated with a bare Awareness. The reason is quite straightforward. Awareness . . . is a featureless sensing or apprehending, and so (by definition) is totally devoid of *all* intrinsic phenomenal characteristics . . .[43]

So much for all those millennia of lab time and the experiences of millions of individuals worldwide. Is it just me, or is the arrogance of modern philosophy sometimes a bit irritating?

Pathological Nothingness

In 2000, a team of psychiatrists at the University of Oklahoma Health Sciences Center reported the case of a ten-year-old boy who claimed he was dead as a result of the 1995 bombing of the Murrah Federal Building, although he was not in Oklahoma City at the time.[44] He furthermore insisted that his grandfather and a friend, and the friend's family, had been killed in the blast, none of which was true.

The child was suffering from a rare condition called Cotard's syndrome, described by the French physician Charles Bonnet in 1788,[45] and later by the Parisian neurologist and psychiatrist Jules Cotard (1840–1889),[46] whose name stuck. The French call the syndrome *délire de négation*.

In its extreme form, the individual has an unshakable belief that he is dead and does not exist. He may believe also that the world outside or parts of it are also nonexistent. Paradoxically, the sufferer may believe he is immortal. In addition, he may become convinced that certain body parts such as the heart, blood, stomach, or intestines are absent, which may lead to self-induced starvation. Convinced that they are dead, Cotard sufferers may smell their flesh rotting or feel maggots or worms crawling through their tissue. This may lead to a request for immediate burial. In fact, Bonnet's first case report involved a woman who insisted on dressing in a burial shroud and being buried. When the authorities refused, she took to a coffin anyway and remained in it until she died weeks later.[47]

Cotard's syndrome occurs in children but usually involves adults. Men and women are affected equally. It appears in the course of schizophrenia and has been reported in brain disorders due to stroke, Alzheimer's disease, brain trauma, temporal lobe epilepsy, and migraine. It responds to psychotropic medications and electroconvulsive therapy.

Cotard's syndrome shows that one can become a nobody through different means. The sense of self and ego can be transcended either through psychospiritual growth or as the result of a malfunctioning brain. The first path leads to joy and fulfillment, the latter to mental illness.

The Vacuum

Scientists used to believe that when empty space was reduced to a vacuum, the result was sheer emptiness or nothing at all. In modern physics, however, the idea of the nothingness has undergone a dramatic transformation. Physicist Harold E. Puthoff, director of the Institute for Advanced Studies in Austin, Texas, describes this shift in thinking and links it to ancient views:

> The metaphysical concept that humanity and the cosmos are interconnected by a ubiquitous, all-pervasive sea of energy that undergirds and is manifest in all phenomena has existed throughout cultural history.
>
> Contemporary physics posits a similar all-pervasive energetic field called "quantum vacuum" or zero-point energy.[48]

Puthoff is the former director of the Cognitive Sciences program at SRI International. During the 1970s, he and fellow-physicist Russell Targ did landmark work in parapsychology, including experiments in remote viewing that seemed to involve the nonlocal transfer of information between distant individuals.[49] Puthoff has long been interested in the eastern idea of *ki* or *chi*, believed to be a universal energy that is involved in such practices as acupuncture and the martial arts. Puthoff suggests that the universal field of chi may essentially be the all-pervasive energetic field of quantum zero-point energy. After all, he wonders, why would nature need *two* universal fields? This would be decidedly "uneconomical." Puthoff suggests that quantum zero-point energy fields, fluctuating throughout the universe, may provide a way for us to be "literally, physically, 'in touch' with the rest of the cosmos." This might be the basis for various non-local manifestations of consciousness, including distant healing, intercessory prayer, and remote knowing. He says,

> [I]f my goal comes to fruition, what will emerge is an under-standing that we are immersed in an overall interpenetrating and interdependent field in ecological balance with the cosmos as a whole. This would dissolve the boundary lines between the phys-ical and "metaphysical" into a unitary viewpoint of the universe as a fluid, changing, energetic/information cosmological unity.[50]

And yet we must be cautious. When mystics speak of the "energy" of consciousness, they are not talking about the sort of stuff that moves a meter on some measuring device. Equating consciousness with zero-point energy or any other physical phenomenon seems to involve a category mistake—confusing the map with the territory or the menu with the meal. But even so, the insights of modern physics make a fan-tastic contribution. As Puthoff explains, they offer a potential explana-tion of how we may be in nonlocal contact with one another, and how information and meaning may be shared remotely between individuals. Along with Puthoff's ideas, several other hypotheses are surfacing from key areas of science that suggest that our oneness with all else is woven into the fabric of the cosmos.[51,52,53,54,55]

Conservation, Prevention, and Placebos

Extracting nonpolluting energy from vacuum fluctuations is currently the holy grail of energy research, and handsome sums are being invested in basic research in this area.[56] There is great irony here—probing invisible space for unlimited energy, when almost all our pre-vious efforts have been focused on the tangible.

Our current national energy policy shows the importance of com-ing to terms with nothing. Consider energy conservation, which was practically reviled during President George W. Bush's first administration. Conservation is an expression of not-doing—not consuming and not wasting. Perhaps policy makers who oppose conservation as a fundamental feature of our national energy policy harbor an underlying horror of not-doing, of emptiness and the void, and project these attitudes onto conservation. When they describe conservationists as do-nothings, they are more correct than they realize, but for the wrong reasons. They are out of touch with the power of nothing, just as classical physicists were blind to the power of the vacuum.

Our society's current energy debate falls into two camps—those who respect and honor nothing and those who fear it. The latter group prefers something over nothing, thus their obsession with expanding the supplies of oil, natural gas, and coal, and building more nuclear power plants. They favor the exploitation of pristine wilderness areas where "nothing ever happens." They are indifferent or actually hostile to alternative sources of energy that resemble nothing, such as the invisible power of the wind and the weightless energy of the sun. On some deep psychological level they seem comforted by the sheer materiality of their favored sources of energy— black oil and black coal. Oil and coal can be seen and held; they are messy, dirty, and physical—the archetypal antithesis of nothing.

In medicine, the analog of conservation is prevention. Like conservation, preventive medicine involves a lot of not-doing, such as avoiding behaviors and habits that lead to disease. To health-care professionals preoccupied with doing, prevention is boring and unglamorous. Effective health care, of course, has always involved equipoise between doing and not-doing. The current problem, however, is that we have so decisively given the upper hand to doing that we have destroyed all balance.

We are astonishingly blind to the consequences of the tyranny of doing. For example, hospital care, our most dramatic form of doing, is currently considered by some experts to be the third leading killer in the United States, behind heart disease and cancer.[57]

A current assault on nothing in medicine involves the placebo response, the power of a fake pill to change the body. Just when the placebo effect appeared to be accepted as a wild card in all therapies, a team of researchers suggested in 2001 that it does not exist.[58] Shortly following this announcement, some observers seemed almost gleeful that the placebo effect had been downgraded to nothing and put in its place.[59] But placebo obituaries are premature. Sophisticated imaging studies have recently shown that when people swallow a placebo, actual physical changes occur in key areas of the brain.[60] These findings clearly show the ability of placebos to tweak tissue.

Alas, the subject of nothing has always inflamed passions. When nothing-related subjects such as spiritual practices, conservation, prevention, and placebos come up, experts invariably line up on both sides—an example of Gibson's Law, the observation that for every Ph.D. there is always an equal and opposite Ph.D.

Drifting Toward Nothing

Most cosmologists believe the universe originated from nothing around 15 billion years ago in the Big Bang, the explosion of "a very hot dot."[61] As the universe cooled, "pieces of vacuum" coalesced, according to physicist John D. Barrow of Cambridge University.[62] These fragments, he says, could have assumed three simple forms—closed loops or infinite lines called cosmic strings; walls or sheets that extend forever; or finite, spherical knots called monopoles.[63] Most physicists currently favor cosmic strings as the best bet.[64]

But when scientists tally up all the known stuff of the universe, they come up short. According to Michael S. Turner,[65] chairman of the department of astronomy and astrophysics at the University of Chicago, 4 percent of the universe is composed of clouds of extremely hot helium and hydrogen gas. A mere 0.5 percent is composed of particles called neutrinos left over from the Big Bang. Another 0.5 percent is the material we ordinarily think of as making up the universe—all the stars in all the galaxies, which includes all the known chemical elements except hydrogen and helium, such as carbon, oxygen, and iron that have formed since the Big Bang in the hearts of stars and in the aftermath of exploding supernovas. That leaves about 95 percent that is invisible—stuff not yet fully identified, which physicists call dark matter and dark energy.

These mystery ingredients are the yin and yang of the universe, says Turner,[66] and their relationship determines the universe's destiny. Dark matter, like all matter, draws mass to it through gravitational pull. This is the tug that allowed matter to combine and form the things we can see—the billions of galaxies and the countless stars they contain. Dark energy, in contrast, operates as a repulsive force, pushing things apart.

Most astronomers currently believe the universe is expanding at an accelerating rate. This means that the repulsive power of dark energy is winning out over the power of dark matter to hold things together. The result is a slide toward a smoothed-out, featureless state in which all matter and energy become diluted and in which all information and complexity are increasingly degraded. Astrophysicists believe the universe will eventually reach a state in which life, as we know it, could not possibly exist.

Amid this dismal scenario, Barrow and other scientists envision various situations that might make possible the perpetuation of life.[67] For instance, the degradation of information is probably not uniform throughout the cosmos. This might permit islands to exist where life in some form might survive. Or perhaps the repulsive force of dark energy will decay in the far future, giving way to the gravitational pull of dark matter. This would allow the aggregation of matter and the processing of information again to become possible, perhaps stoking the furnace of life. Or perhaps our descendants will master techniques by which they can control runaway acceleration in their vicinity of the universe and engineer life-enhancing outcomes.

Or perhaps the universe will reproduce itself and start all over. Although Barrow considers this unlikely, he adds, "When we have an infinite future to worry about all this, fantastically improbable physical occurrences will eventually have a significant chance of occurring. . . . When there is an infinite time to wait then *anything* that can happen, eventually *will* happen. Worse (or better) than that, it will happen infinitely often."[68] But even if the universe begins anew, Barrow believes this holds little comfort for human life. "Globally," he says, "the self-reproduction may inspire new beginnings, new physics, new dimensions, but, along our world line, in our part of the Universe, there will ultimately be sameness, starless and lifeless, forever, it seems. Perhaps it's good that we won't be there after all."[69]

Depressed about this one-way descent into nothing? So, too, is Woody Allen, who lamented, "More than any other time in history, mankind faces a crossroads. One path leads to despair and utter hopelessness. The other, to total extinction. Let us pray we have the wisdom to choose correctly."[70]

Yet it is far too early to cede the future to the prophets of cosmic doom and to nothingness. Science hasn't had the last word, it has hardly had the first word on what this nothing, into which we are supposed to be sliding, actually is.

In discussions of the origin and destiny of the universe, the role of consciousness—the greatest unknown in all of science—is usually left out. An exception is the work of the eminent physicist John Archibald Wheeler, who believes that "we are a part of a universe that is a work in progress; we are tiny patches of the universe looking at itself—and building itself . . . a clue that the mystery of creation may lie not in the distant past but in the living present."[71] Stanford University physicist Andrei Linde agrees that consciousness is an essential factor in the universe. "The universe and the observer exist as a pair," he says. "We are together, the universe and us. . . . I cannot imagine a consistent theory of everything that ignores consciousness."[72]

A plethora of evidence suggests that consciousness is genuinely nonlocal or infinite, lying beyond the space and time in which our bodies are embedded, and therefore immune to degradation by the universe's expansion.[73]

So to those who may be forlorn about our fate in the far cosmic future, I advise dwelling on the nonlocal, infinite nature of consciousness. Think of it this way: The implication of nonlocal mind is immortality, in which nothing and nobody are revealed as everything, everywhere, and forever.

Not a bad consolation prize.

12

Voices

Out of the air a voice without a face . . .

—*W. H. AUDEN, "The Shield of Achilles"*

One of the most low-tech health methodologies in human history is the hearing of voices. This is a broad-spectrum therapy, affecting physical and mental health alike.

In the sixth century BCE, Epimenedes went into prolonged trances, and on coming out of them told how conversations with the spirits gave him advice on a variety of problems, including how to ward off a threatened plague.[1] The oracles in ancient Greece did the same, often dispensing instructions on how to avoid plagues and epidemics.

Moses took verbal orders that influenced the physical, psychological, and spiritual health of his people, spoken to him both directly from God or indirectly, as through the burning bush. A contemporary Bush, President George W., also says he receives information from his "higher father."[2] Although the president does not say he actually hears voices, the instructions he receives, like the voice Moses heard, profoundly affect the health of his people and that of millions around the world, bearing as they do on issues such as war, poverty, AIDS, pollution, and global warming.

Socrates communicated with his daemon or inner spirit for hours at a time. He suggested that in order to make the most of voices it helps to be a little crazy. "The greatest blessings come by way of madness, if it is heaven sent," he told Phaedrus. "It was when they were mad that the prophetesses at Delphi and the priestesses at Dodona achieved so much; . . . when sane they did little or nothing." Flirting with madness paradoxically yielded benefits for one's mental health. Letting the voices come through unburdened an individual, relieved him of his troubles, and opened a doorway to the muses, who made one more creative. The great poets, Socrates said, "do not attain to excellence through the rules of any art; they utter their beautiful verses in a state of inspiration."[3]

The difficulty, now as then, lies in knowing whether or not the voice we hear is truly "heaven sent." The recipient is just as important as the source, for raving madmen also hear voices, and they may garble the message even when it is genuine. And even if the voices do originate in heaven and are received intact, that is no guarantee they are benign, for, as the Greeks were aware, the gods sometimes play tricks and drive men insane. As Hera warned in *The Iliad,* "The gods are hard to cope with, when seen very clearly . . ."[4]

Voices are notoriously ambiguous. An example of double-talking voices is given by Herodotus—the fall of Croesus's Lydian Empire in 546 BCE.[5] Croesus was uncertain whether he should allow Cyrus of Persia to continue to build up his military forces, or crush them with a sudden preemptive strike. In a controlled trial that sounds quite modern, Croesus sent out envoys to each of the best-known oracles, asking them what he would be doing at a specific hour on a particular day. The oracle at Delphi replied, "The savour of the hard-shelled tortoise, boiled in brass with the flesh of lamb, strikes on my senses. Brass is laid beneath it, and brass is put over it." Croesus, at the appointed hour, had in fact cut up a lamb and tortoise and boiled them in a brass kettle. This reply emboldened him to ask the Delphic oracle the next question: Should he attack Cyrus? The reply was,

When Croesus has the Halys crossed
A mighty Empire will be lost.

Believing he had received a divine imprimatur to go ahead, Croesus attacked and was defeated, thus fulfilling the oracle's prediction that a mighty empire would fall. Those in our day who see God's will in preemptive war might ponder this example.

For all the challenges voices present, it is vital for our mental health to keep the channels open, because when the voices of the gods are shut out those of the devils often take up residence. Something of this sort seems to have happened during the evolution of Christianity. By the medieval period, voices and visions were largely suspected as pagan and demonic. The criteria that arose to discriminate the divine from the satanic versions were stringent even for the saintly, and for the common person voices were all but banished. As the old avenues—one of which was dreams—were closed, a price was paid. As religion scholar Jacques Le Goff puts it, "With the path of dreams blocked, the way was open for nightmares . . . medieval man would not re-conquer the dream-world for a long time to come."[6] One of the nightmares that arose, Le Goff states, was that of purgatory, the stopping-off place where the soul was indefinitely stranded until one's sins were expiated.

What differentiates a hallucinating schizophrenic from a Socrates? This question has never been easy to answer. The Greek historian Plutarch, who as far as we know did not hear voices, took a dim view of Socrates's chattering daemon. He maintained that the spirits had no need to be vociferous in order to convey information. "We may surmise," he said, speaking of Socrates's vocal spirit, "that what reached him was not a voice or a sound, but the silent voice of the daemon, touching the intelligence of his soul. . . . [Daemons] need neither the names nor the words which men use in speaking to one another, to put across their ideas."[7]

The ancient Greeks were convinced voices could assist in healing, and they courted them in their healing temples or *asklepions.* Greek healers invented ways of facilitating dreams in their patients as well as themselves, in which the goal was often to dream of not only the diagnosis but the proper therapy as well.

Medical assistance from voices or spirits may seem quaint, but still occurs. Barbara Stevens Barnum, PhD, RN, former editor of *Nursing & Health Care* and author of *Mystic Encounters: The Door Ajar*,[8] has researched nurses' experiences of what she calls "expanded consciousness"— events that can't be explained rationally and which appear to transcend the physical senses. In a survey of 121 nurse leaders, all of whom held doctorates or master's degrees, she found that 41 percent of them described such experiences.

One of these outstanding nurses described an event that took place a year after her husband died.[9] She remarried, and she and her new husband were cleaning the backyard of an old farmhouse they had rented. As she was picking up armloads of rotten, termite-infested lumber without gloves, she heard her deceased husband's voice say, in his Cajun accent, "Don't—step back—there's a rattler under there." She picked up the next layer of rotten boards with a pitchfork, saw the rattlesnake, and killed it. "Thank you," she said to her deceased husband. Two days later she revisited the site and saw him standing there. "No one can ever convince me this experience did not happen," she said. "I'm sane, mature, adult, productive, creative, active and *normal.* I only wish I knew how to be more receptive and to have more control over my 'extra' sense."

Scary? In Barnum's survey, "not one account mentioned fear or dread; on the contrary, many described the comfort of the contact [with the deceased individual]."[10]

Experiences such as these are universal. When bereavement researcher W. D. Rees interviewed 227 widows and 66 widowers, he found that nearly half of them had "visitation experiences" from the deceased, almost 15 percent of which took the form of spoken messages. These experiences involved both sexes, cut across every culture, were common in small villages and large cities, and happened to agnostics, atheists, and believers alike.[11]

Hearing voices can be healthy, say psychiatric researchers Marius Romme and Sandra Escher, authors of *Making Sense of Voices*.[12] "It is clear that just because you hear voices does not necessarily mean you should be diagnosed with schizophrenia or even that you have a mental health problem," they say. How to tell the difference? For Romme and Escher, voices are a problem only when the person has difficulty coping with them, or when the experience impinges on the lives of others.[13] Their conclusions are reinforced by their study of 15,000 people living in Baltimore, nearly 2,000 of whom heard voices. This amounts to around fifteen percent of the population—far greater than the percentage believed to be schizophrenic, unless there is something strangely amiss in Baltimore.[14]

There may be an evolutionary reason why we hear voices. Human beings need contact with others, and research shows that those who enjoy rich social connections live longer and are healthier than those who live in isolation. Do voices appear in order to keep us company? Are they a device to counteract the unhealthy effects of loneliness? If so, they would constitute survival value for the individual and would tend to be internalized as a part of our genetic makeup and be passed down to succeeding generations.

Psychologist Julian Jaynes offers a possible mechanism for voices in his provocative book *The Origin of Consciousness in the Breakdown of the Bicameral Mind*.[15] He suggests that, in our early evolutionary history, cross-talking voices from the two sides of our brain were the norm. The result was a two-way conversation that today would be regarded as a schizophrenic dialogue. Our right and left cerebral hemispheres became differently specialized, Jaynes suggests, as a way of quieting this interhemispheric babble.

Regardless of how and why voices originated, we should not romanticize them because they are not always benign. As transpersonal psychologist Arthur Hastings states in his admirable book *With the Tongues of Men and Angels*, voices often make critical comments to normal people that are actually objective and accurate, but which can be challenging and unpleasant.[16] Psychopaths often describe being guided by voices telling them to take revenge or to murder someone. There is the danger, too, that people will play fast and loose with voices in order to justify their actions. This is particularly true with world leaders and governments. As we've seen, President George W. Bush claims divine guidance in waging war and fighting terrorism.[17] His arch-enemy, Osama bin Laden, claims his god provides him with similar messages, but directed against Mr. Bush. Religious leaders, both Christian and Islamic, have questioned the interpretations of both men.[18]

Musical Voices

"Voices" imply that someone is speaking, but of course voices sing, too. Very little attention has been paid to musical voices or what clinical psychiatrists call musical auditory hallucinations. In a rare study at Pittsburgh's Western Psychiatric Institute and Clinic, however, researchers P. R. Saba and M. S. Keshavan questioned one hundred consecutive schizophrenic inpatients about the presence of musical hallucinations and musical imagery. Sixteen responded positively. The music that was most frequently associated with these experiences was religious in nature.[19]

Music also invades the minds of normal people, against their will. Everyone has had the experience of having a tune stick in the mind so tightly it seems impossible to stop thinking about it. James Kellaris, a professor at University of Cincinnati, calls this experience the Stuck Tune Syndrome, and he is trying to figure out why it happens.[20] The syndrome is like a "cognitive itch," he says—a musical mosquito bite, in which the more you scratch the more agonizing it becomes.

Scholars suggest that stuck tunes may be a positive factor in mental health. Diana Deutsch, a leading musicologist and psychology professor at UC-San Diego, says that tunes get stuck for a reason. Whenever they won't go away, something in the back of our mind is trying to tell us something. When we've got the message, we may hang up the phone. How? Whenever she has this experience she contemplates the meaning of the lyrics, and the song instantly disappears.[21]

In 2001, Kellaris reported the results of interviews of one thousand students at four universities, and found that almost all the students reported having endured songs or jingles they could not stop thinking about. Although 55 percent said the typical episode lasted only a few hours, 23 percent said it remained for a full day. Seventeen percent described the problem persisting several days, and 5 percent said it lasted longer than a week. One unfortunate individual claimed that a tune from an Atari 260 video game had been humming in his head since 1986. Kellaris identified three key characteristics of the stickiest songs—excessive repetition, musical simplicity, and incongruity, in which the beat or lyric defies the listener's expectations.

In and of themselves, stuck tunes are not healing, which is the theme of this book. But once they're there, there are a few things you can do to dislodge them. As a recurrent sufferer from stuck tunes, I've discovered that Deutsch's recommendation to contemplate the tune's meaning does not always vanquish it. So it doesn't surprise me that Kellaris's students reported a variety of additional methods to heal themselves of the malignant melody. The most common was to think of another tune to subvert and drive out the offending one. Some remedies were rooted in folklore; one student chewed a cinnamon stick and swore it had a 100 percent success rate. Others simply distracted themselves by focusing on another task.

The top ten offending tunes Kellaris discovered were (WARNING: You may want to skip this):

1. "The Macarena"
2. "I'm a Little Teacup"
3. Theme from *Gilligan's Island*
4. Chili's baby-back ribs jingle
5. "1812 Overture" by Tchaikovsky
6. "The Gambler" by Kenny Rogers

7. "YMCA"

8. Two Dr. Pepper jingles

9. "Eine Kleine Nachtmusik" by Mozart

10. Themes from *The Andy Griffith Show* and *The Odd Couple*

Extraordinary Voices

Sometimes voices seem downright benevolent.

In the winter of 1984, a woman I'll call Annie heard a distinct voice in her head while sitting in her London home reading. It said, "Please don't be afraid. I know it must be shocking for you to hear me speaking like this, but this is the easiest way I could think of. My friend and I used to work at Children's Hospital, Great Ormond Street, and we would like to help you." Thus began one of the most remarkable case reports ever published in the prestigious *British Medical Journal*,[22] and a profound example of the extraordinary healing power of ordinary things.

Annie was born in Europe in the mid-1940s and settled in Britain in the late 1960s. She worked at a series of jobs, married, had children, and devoted herself to being a housewife and mother. She was completely healthy, as far as she knew, and had never required hospital treatment.

Although she had heard of Children's Hospital, which the voice mentioned, she did not know where it was. Her children were healthy and she had never needed the services of such a hospital, so the message was confusing. The voice spoke again: "To help you see that we are sincere, we would like you to check out the following," and gave her three separate items of information unknown to her at the time, which she confirmed as true. By this time Annie was convinced that she was going mad. In a state of panic, she visited her personal physician, who sent her immediately to a psychiatrist.

It was a fortunate referral. Dr. Ikechukwu O. Azuonye, a consulting psychiatrist who was a graduate of the University of Nigeria School of Medicine, diagnosed her as having a "functional hallucinatory psychosis." He began counseling and thioridazine, an antipsychotic medication. By the end of two weeks the voices had disappeared. Annie was so relieved she went on vacation to celebrate. But while abroad, still taking her medication, the voices reappeared. They instructed her to return to England immediately. Something was wrong with her, they said, which required urgent treatment. Other beliefs also began flooding her mind at this time, which were obviously delusional.

Quite upset, she aborted her holiday and returned to England and saw Dr. Azuonye again. Now the voices gave Annie a specific address to go to. Her husband, just to reassure her that "it was all in her mind," reluctantly drove her there. The address turned out to be the computerized tomography department of a large London hospital. On arrival, the voices told her to go inside and request a brain scan because she had a tumor in her brain. Because the information the voices provided earlier had proved true, Annie believed them.

In order to relieve her fears, Dr. Azuonye ordered a brain scan. He told the radiologists about the voices and their diagnostic message, and acknowledged that there was no physical evidence for a brain tumor. The request for the scan was denied. The radiologists implied that Dr. Azuonye had gone overboard, was squandering medical resources and driving up costs, and had been taken in by his patient's delusions. When Dr. Azuonye persisted, the radiologists relented and performed the scan. They were alarmed at the findings and did a repeat procedure, which confirmed a large brain tumor. Dr. Azuonye referred Annie to a neurosurgeon, who suggested an immediate operation. The voices agreed, telling Annie that this was the correct decision. At surgery, a tumor was found in the left frontal area, extending to the right side. It was removed completely and proved to be a meningioma, which is not metastatic and invasive, but which can kill by compressing adjacent brain structures.

When Annie regained consciousness after surgery the voices announced, "We are pleased to have helped you. Goodbye." She recovered uneventfully without complications. Her antipsychotic medication was stopped following the operation, and the voices did not return.

Dr. Azuonye set the case aside. But twelve years later, when Annie phoned him at Christmas to wish him and his family a merry festive season, he felt he had an obligation to report this unusual case.

In his 1997 write-up in the *British Medical Journal*, Dr. Azuonye reports that this is the only instance he has been able to identify in which "hallucinatory voices" reassured a patient of their interest, offered a specific diagnosis in the total absence of physical signs and symptoms, directed the patient to the address of the specific type of hospital needed to diagnose the problem, expressed pleasure that the treatment they desired was successful, bid farewell, and quietly and completely quit the scene.

The previous year, in 1996, Dr. Azuonye had presented her case at a hospital conference. He had invited Annie to attend, and she had been questioned by several physicians in the audience. The doctors were evenly divided in their reactions. One group was what Dr. Azuonye called the X-philes, who rejoiced in Annie's good fortune and believed she had received genuine telepathic communication from the voices seeking to help her. Then there were the X-phobes, those physicians who could not accept voices. Their favored explanation was that it was a hoax. They suggested that Annie had originally learned of her diagnosis in her native country and invented the voices in order to obtain free treatment in Britain from the National Health Service. Yet Annie had lived in Britain for fifteen years and was already entitled to NHS treatment. In addition, she was panicked by the voices and was so overjoyed when they vanished after initial treatment with thioridazine that she went on holiday to celebrate regaining her sanity. Other skeptics suggested a scenario involving her unconscious mind. Even though the tumor did not cause overt symptoms, the skeptics said she must have had some sensation from it, which led to the fear of a brain tumor and to her hallucination of voices. She must have unconsciously known more about the hospital than she realized, and attributed this information to the voices. The goodbye message was her unconscious mind speaking, signifying her relief that things had worked out well. Others suggested that, since the voices originated with the brain tumor and went away with its surgical removal, this obviously indicated that the tumor was the source of the voices.

This case report is noteworthy not only for the voices themselves, but also because it reveals the lengths skeptics go to in order to dismiss voices as hallucinations or lies: Consciousness is defended as individual, private, and personal, something that is derived from one's brain and confined to it. Consciousness is not a party line. Individual minds are sealed off from all other minds, and voices can't chime in.

Where Is Consciousness?

If you hear a voice out of the clear blue and tell people about it, you can be certain they will doubt your sanity and regard you as having a "condition" of some sort. As comedienne Lily Tomlin said, "When we talk to God we are praying; when God talks to us, we are schizophrenic."[23]

Tomlin's right; we have pathologized "voices." But the voices haven't gotten the message, and they keep turning up in the experiences of normal individuals.[24] If you don't hear voices, you could be in the minority. Surveys show that up to half of a non-clinical population has hallucinatory experiences such as voices at least once a month.[25,26] That's a lot of chatter, and a lot of people are keeping quiet about it.

Voices are particularly frequent in individuals who live on the creative edge. A friend who is a well-known artist carries on a continual conversation with "them." She can hardly complete a sentence without referring to what "they" told her, "they" being her "angelic guides from another dimension." Most individuals who hear voices react similarly, attributing them to a specific entity of some sort— guardians, guides, angels, saints, ancestors, or spirits.

Why can't we let a voice be just a voice? Why assign it to a specific person and place? This reflects the way we think about our own consciousness, which most people feel is located in their head in the midline about an inch or so behind the eyes. For Nobel physicist Erwin

Schrödinger, this ingrained (or inbrained) way of thinking is entirely arbitrary.[27] Consciousness, he maintained, is not in a precise anatomical or geographic location, but can be anywhere. Some cultures have assigned it not to the head but to the heart, chest, or abdomen. Consciousness, suggested Schrödinger, may even be outside the body. A neurosurgeon colleague of mine agrees. He says that when he operates his consciousness is not inside his cranium but is at the tip of his scalpel. It goes ahead, runs interference, and tells him what to cut and what to avoid.

Yet when people hear voices, they assume they must be coming from an embodied entity somewhat like ourselves. A voice, like consciousness, requires a body, which we trick out as an angel or alien, god or devil.

Voices and History

Human history has been dramatically shaped by voices. Subtract voices, and the course of world affairs is hardly interpretable. Examples abound in all the world's major religions, such as God thundering to Moses on Mt. Sinai or Allah revealing the Koran to Mohammed. The Vedas, the oldest Hindu scriptures, are poetic hymns heard by sages. Tibetan Buddhist teachers over the centuries claim to have received teachings directly from deities and other discarnate beings. Many scriptures in Taoism have been received by direct revelation. In politics and governance we see a similar pattern. For centuries the Delphic oracle inspired and guided the ancient Greeks in enacting laws, planning wars and battles, exploring, plotting trade routes, and understanding the causes of plagues and famines. In fifteenth-century France, a divine voice inspired Joan of Arc to help restore the crown to Charles VII and defeat the invading English forces, which proved the turning point in the Hundred Years' War.[28] Florence Nightingale heard the voice of God repeatedly, leading her to found modern secular nursing and advance public health throughout the world.[29]

Educator Alfred Alschuler has assembled 150 significant individuals in history who heard voices that provided healing, worthy information, and inspiration. They include persons such as Martin Luther, St. Teresa of Avila, and Winston Churchill, whose life was saved when he heard an inner voice telling him to move to the other side of his car just before a bomb exploded on the side where he had been. Voices often appear neutral with respect to whom they help. They may have saved Churchill, but during World War I a voice also told a young Adolf Hitler to move down a trench just before a shell exploded, killing everyone in the group where he was sitting.[30,31,32]

Opening Up: Lessons from Transplants

Sometimes voices are muted in health situations, appearing as urges and inclinations rather than spoken words.

In 1988, Claire Sylvia, a professional dancer, underwent a successful heart-and-lung transplant at Yale-New Haven Hospital.[33] She got more than new organs. While recovering from surgery, Sylvia developed a craving for foods she had never liked before, such as beer, green peppers, and chicken nuggets. She became convinced that this had something to do with her donor, and that he was trying to communicate with her. A friend of hers dreamed that her donor was an 18-year-old man who had been killed in a motorcycle accident. This information enabled her to trace her donor's identity and meet his family. They confirmed that Sylvia's new food preferences were those of the deceased donor. Her story is described in her 1997 book *A Change of Heart: A Memoir.* When her story was picked up by the media and featured on *60 Minutes*, this encouraged other transplant recipients to come forward with similar revelations.

Skeptics attribute these events to mere coincidence and an overheated imagination. Proponents, on the other hand, usually invoke "cellular memory" as an explanation. This is the idea that our thoughts are somehow encoded in our tissues, and that if our organs are transplanted into someone else, something of our emotional life is transferred along with them. Yet there is no evidence that any cell in the body can actually store a specific thought, nor any known way in which this might happen. True, when neuroscientists stimulate specific areas of the brain, certain thoughts may appear in the mind of the individual, suggesting they must be stored in brain cells. However, this does not prove that thoughts reside in brain tissue any more than an image on the television screen is proof that the image lives in the TV set. Attributing transplant-related mental phenomena to transferred organs reflects the need to dress up thoughts in something physical, in the same way we need to assign voices to some sort of entity.

Blood transfusions are a kind of transplant and have been done millions of times. Surgeons have also performed thousands of kidney transplants over decades. If cellular memory is real and if thoughts are transferable via cells and tissues, why has this phenomenon only recently been noticed?

It is easy to see how we might be misled on this point. Imagine a battery-powered television set plopped down into a remote jungle, whose inhabitants have had no prior contact with civilization. When the TV is turned on and images of people appear on the screen, the natives would think they originated in the box itself. How could they think otherwise, having no concept of invisible electromagnetic signals being bounced off satellites in space?

In the same way, when we witness an organ transplanted into a body, and all of a sudden new thoughts and traits appear in the recipient, it is natural to think that they, too, originated in the transplanted organ. But this may be as erroneous as supposing that television images reside in the TV set itself. Breaking out of this mode of thinking requires a shift, in which we begin to think of consciousness as infinite or nonlocal, instead of being confined to cells, tissues, and organs.

It is possible that human bodies act as focusing devices for information that is spread throughout the universe, just as mechanical devices such as television sets and radios focus invisible electromagnetic signals. Certain parts of human bodies—especially brains—are quite adept at focusing information, although why this is so is a mystery.

I therefore doubt that the donated organ possesses "cellular memory" of the donor's experiences, which are then decoded or played back in the recipient following the transplant. This "cassette theory"—in which the donated organ is the cassette tape containing the information, and the recipient's body is the cassette player that decodes or plays back the information—reflects a longing for physical explanations we can see and touch. I believe a better explanation is that consciousness is not in a place in space or time, but is what I've called *nonlocal mind*.[34] "Nonlocal" is just a fancy word for infinite. Nonlocal, boundless mind would permit the consciousness of the donor to be fundamentally united with the consciousness of the recipient, enabling Claire Sylvia to gain information about her donor.

How common are nonlocal experiences among transplant recipients? No one knows. As it becomes more acceptable to talk about them, we may find that post-transplant experiences such as Claire Sylvia's occur more frequently than we think.

It is a mistake to consider these experiences new. Organ transplantation may be modern, but nonlocal awareness isn't. Voices are part of our human legacy, and they are not yet done with us.

Avenues of Awareness

Throughout history human beings have discovered a variety of ways to experience their nonlocal connections with others. Sometimes physical objects serve this purpose. A ring, locket, photo, or lock of hair helps lovers realize their unity in spite of physical separation. They know that the physical object doesn't actually contain the other person, but is a symbol that triggers unifying associations in the consciousness of the two individuals. A part of the body—a donated heart or kidney or lung—might function symbolically in the same way.

Marie-Louise von Franz, a close collaborator of Carl Jung, describes a village in the Swiss canton of Uri where the church and cemetery are on the other side of a little river. In a funeral, they have to carry the coffin over the bridge that leads to the church and cemetery. A dry mud path leads to the bridge, and in good weather the mud cracks. As people follow the coffin, they stare at the chaotic pattern of the cracks in the dry mud, and they claim that this reveals to them who will be the next person to die. This experience, associated as it is with life and death, "delocalizes" their consciousness, so to speak, and makes access to future information possible.

So it may be with transplant recipients who take on the behaviors and thoughts of their donors. The life-and-death nature of the transplant experience may free their minds, so they have access to what a deceased donor thought or dreamed, how he behaved, and, in Claire Sylvia's case, what he liked for lunch.

Von Franz describes how she once consulted a famous Dutch palmist named Spier who had written a book on the subject. Spier read palms with a twist. He put soot on the client's palm, made an imprint on paper, and read from that. But von Franz would not let him read her future. "I thought I owned my own future and that was none of his business," she stated, "so I [allowed him] only to tell me my past." Von Franz, a natural skeptic and one of the keenest observers in the history of modern psychology, described Spier's revelations of her past as "fantastic." Intrigued, she arranged to have coffee with him and pressed him to reveal how he did it. He maintained that he was a genuine medium and that when a person came into his consulting room he simply knew all about them, although he could not explain how. The sole purpose of the performance with the soot and the lines and cracks on the palm was to liberate the unconscious knowledge he already possessed, so he could make it known to his client. Von Franz explains:

The unconscious *knows* things; it knows the past and future, it knows things about other people. We all from time to time have dreams which inform us about something which happens to another person. . . . A medium is a person who has one might say a gift, by which to relate to the absolute knowledge of the unconscious, generally by having a relatively low level of consciousness. This explains why mediums are very often very queer and often even morally odd people—not always, but often—or they are slightly criminal, or take a drink, and so on. They are generally very endangered personalities because they have that low threshold and are so near to the absolute knowledge of the unconscious.[35]

The experience of serious illness, which having an organ transplant surely is, may lower the threshold of consciousness, as von Franz describes, allowing the influx of thoughts that are normally screened out, including nonlocal contact with the thoughts and traits of the donor. This can be unsettling and disturbing, as the experience of voices was to Annie, and may require psychiatric care. As organ transplantation becomes more common, we may see the emergence of a new field—transplantation psychiatry—to help recipients deal with these problems. If the new counselors are to be effective, they will need to be well-versed in the principles of nonlocal, infinite mind, as Dr. Azuonye, Annie's psychiatrist, seemed to have been.

"We could all be mediums, and all have absolute knowledge, if the bright light of our ego consciousness would not dim it," von Franz states. "That is why the medium needs . . . to go into a trance, a sleep-like state, to pull up his or her knowledge. I have myself observed that in states of extreme fatigue, when I am really dangerously physically exhausted, I suddenly get absolute knowledge; I am much closer to it then, but as soon as I have slept well for a few nights then this wonderful gift is gone again. Why? Absolute knowledge is like candlelight, and if the electric light of ego consciousness is burning, then one cannot see the candlelight."[36]

Pre-modern cultures devised ways of dimming the light of consciousness in order for nonlocal knowledge to emerge. One Native

American technique was the vision quest, in which a young man ventured into a remote area, fasted without food or water for days, exposed himself to predation by wild animals, and became exhausted and sleep-deprived. He often had a vision of his future—the life he should lead, how he should contribute to the welfare of his tribe, and his mode of death.

My internship and residency in internal medicine was a three-year exercise in sleep deprivation and physical fatigue, in essence a protracted vision quest. Sometimes I felt I was functioning more dead than alive. Although I shudder to think of the mistakes I made, I was nonetheless freeing up avenues into my unconscious mind without realizing it. We physicians like to complain about the rigors of our profession, but some of us realize at an unconscious level that sleep deprivation and chronic fatigue can sometimes play valuable roles.

After practicing internal medicine for over a decade, I proposed to the internists in my medical group a method whereby we could relieve our nighttime on-call duties and guarantee regular sleep, rest, and renewal. Several of my fellow physicians were actually offended by the proposal and it was soundly defeated. One young internist said adamantly, "Night call is what doctors do. We *need* night call!" I considered this unalloyed stubbornness at the time, but perhaps he was more correct than I realized. Taking away sleep deprivation and chronic fatigue, as onerous as they are, might erase an avenue into nonlocal awareness. It might interfere with nonlocal approaches to making diagnoses and formulating treatments, which my colleagues may have dimly sensed.

Physicians flirt with methods to expand awareness without realizing it. Psychiatrists ask their patients to stare at Rorschach blots, which liberate the unconscious mind. Radiologists stare at X-rays in dimly lit rooms, and are sometimes called "shadow gazers" by us nonradiologists. I know radiologists who are so skillful in discerning meaningful patterns on X-rays that they seem almost clairvoyant.

Voices throughout history have assisted healing by bringing comfort and consolation and by offering advice in managing medical problems, as we've seen. Where have they gone? You'd leave too, if those you spoke to never listened and pretended you did not exist.

Although I have experienced prophetic dreams with specific medical content, I have never heard voices. I often wonder why. Perhaps my daemon is not talkative because it "needs neither the names nor the words which men use," as Plutarch said, to get the points across. Or perhaps I'm simply not listening. Perhaps I carry more unconscious resistance to voices than I realize, having become biased against them in the course of my medical education. Whatever the reason, I envy my voice-hearing physician predecessors in ancient Greece, who were tapped into channels of information that seemed to flow directly from the Source.

Although I lament their absence, I have to admit that hearing voices is not exactly the best way to advance one's career in medicine these days. Admitting one does so is likely to get one sanctioned, medicated, and locked up.

I belong to the profession that has adopted the most hostile stance toward voices since the Middle Ages. Over the past 2,500 years, the pendulum of disbelief in voices held by medicine has swung as far in one direction as it can possibly go. Today, physicians reject not only the accuracy of voices, but also any source of wisdom from which they *could* originate. We insist that the only source of medical wisdom is our own minds via the logical analysis we bring to bear on a problem. There is no outside Source to help us. We are on our own. Yet, disbelief is only half of it. We have also become overtaken by a paranoid obsession to pathologize voices, extinguish them through every means possible, and stigmatize those who hear them. The most reasonable explanation for this crusade against voices is fear. We are scared out of our wits that there may be "something else" out there, that we are not in total control.

The ancient Greeks would have considered our refusal of the help offered by voices as dangerously arrogant. They would have said that our denial of a Source outside ourselves amounts to hubris. And they would have predicted our downfall, for that is the punishment the gods reserve for those who adopt such prideful positions.

Lately, I have begun asking for the voices to return to medicine, to physicians, to me, and that when they do, we have the great good sense to listen. I know this is dangerous turf, and that "when the gods want to punish us, they answer our prayers." Still, we need all the wisdom we can lay hold of, regardless of where it comes from.

We have lost our way in our profession by denying the existence of any variety of mind other than that which exists above the clavicles and between the ears of the highest primate. May the gods forgive us—and resume the conversation we once had.

13

Mystery

I am entirely on the side of the mystery.
I mean, any attempts to explain away the mystery is
ridiculous. . . . I believe in the profound and unfathomable mystery
of life . . . which has a . . . divine quality about it. . . .

—ALDOUS HUXLEY

When I applied to medical school many years ago, I was asked to write an essay on "Why I Want to Be a Doctor." I focused on relieving human suffering, as pre-med students usually do when faced with this question. My paper plus good grades worked, and I was accepted to the medical school of my choice. But I was being less than truthful in the essay. I wasn't primarily attracted to medicine because of an altruistic impulse. I was hooked on mystery.

I was particularly enchanted by physiology and biochemistry as an undergraduate. I wondered how the brain of a human being could "make" consciousness, which I was assured brains did. As I pursued a degree in pharmacy, I encountered the fascinating field of pharmacognosy, the study of medicinal plants. The fact that a molecule derived from a crude plant could alter one's consciousness and for a while radically shift one's world view seemed pure magic. How could the actions of a physical substance translate into something that seems completely nonphysical, like thought? Questions of this sort were never discussed. These mysteries were so deep they seemed taboo. I assumed they would be addressed in medical school, but I found that they continued to be ignored there, too.

During medical school I was drawn to internal medicine, which is all about solving mysteries. The foundation of internal medicine is *diagnosis*—from the Latin *dia* and *gnosis*, "a knowing that exists between or through two people." Internists, it seemed to me, were individuals who passionately wanted to *know* things, specifically the identity of the patient's illness and how to treat it. Internists, more than any other type of physician, found delight in mystery. That's why our surgery-leaning colleagues, whose infatuation lay more in doing than in knowing, derided us internal medicine-oriented students as "swamis" and "crystal-ball gazers."[1]

When a patient comes to a physician with a medical problem, it has no label. Diagnosis is the art of sorting out a single answer from many possibilities. The gateway to diagnosis is mystery. Mystery and knowing embrace each other in a complex dance, each sustaining the other: Without mystery there is nothing to know; without knowing, the concept of mystery does not arise.

The diagnosis of a complicated illness always involves a list of possibilities, which psychologist William James called "maybes." For me, sorting out the maybes in an individual case transcended dry intellectualizing. Diseases weren't just chapters in medical textbooks, they were experienced by real people as pain, suffering, fear, and despair. Internists were bound by oath to help resolve these difficulties and restore hope and health. Making sense of all the maybes was the key to this task, to which I decided to devote my life. This mission related to not only patients but to my own journey in life as well, which, like everyone's path, involves an endless string of choices among a cloud of maybes. As James wisely put it, "[S]o far as man stands for anything, and is productive and originative at all, his entire vital function may be said to have to deal with maybes. Not a victory is gained, not a deed of faithfulness or courage is done, except upon a maybe."[2]

I often wondered why some of my fellow students chose "doing" fields such as orthopedics, urology, or neurosurgery, while others selected "knowing" areas such as internal medicine and psychiatry. At the time, I attributed these choices to individual temperament and let it go at that. Eventually, however, I began to realize that a key influence pushing young doctors into various specialties was their differing attitudes towards mystery.

Tolerance for ambiguity and mystery helps explain many of the directions I've taken—not only internal medicine but also the field of complementary-alternative therapies, the role of spirituality and consciousness in health, and my editorship of the medical journal *Explore*, whose very name suggests the unknowns that lie over the horizon.

In addition to mystery, I'm certain there are other factors pushing me in these directions that I only dimly perceive. I've even wondered about the influence of one's name on one's choices—what's been called "nominative determinism," suggested by orthopedists who are evocatively named "Bone," urologists named "Water," and cardiologists named "Hart."[3] Flip a couple of letters and add a "y," and Dossey becomes "Odyssey," a long series of travels, adventures, and encounters with mystery.

Mystery and Health

Our hunger for the mysterious is more than curiosity. Mystery is vital to our physical, mental, and spiritual health.

Dr. Marilyn Albert, chair of the medical and scientific council of the Alzheimer's Association, emphasizes ways of preventing Alzheimer's disease and the cognitive decline that accompanies aging. "The brain is more plastic than we thought," she says. "It has the capacity to renew and regenerate. . . ."[4]

Some of the factors that help preserve mental function into old age are extraordinarily simple. In a study in Finland of 1,500 elderly people, those who were obese in middle age were twice as likely to develop dementia in old age as those who were of normal weight. For those who had high blood pressure and high cholesterol in middle age, their risk was six times greater than those not having these problems in mid-life. In another study involving 13,000 women, those who ate vegetables such as spinach, lettuce, broccoli, and Brussels sprouts in middle age preserved more of their mental faculties as they entered their 70s, compared to women who ate fewer vegetables. Physical exercise and social involvement were also related to better cognitive function. But the discovery that surprised many was that mental activities like reading books and problem solving, such as doing crossword puzzles and playing bingo, were also found to help prevent mental decline. What other activities might work? "Anything," Albert says, "that will push people to encounter something that isn't routine."

Routines are ruts, and they become deeper the longer we stay in them. Getting out of them isn't easy, because they provide predictability, comfort, and security. Routines don't require much brainpower; we generally know what's coming next. When we rupture routines we experience uncertainty, which—key step—permits a bit of mystery to seep into our life. When mystery kicks in, we are no longer on automatic pilot; we have to *think*. Perhaps this is why mystery is good for the brain: Mystery places demands on it, and the brain, being "more plastic than we thought," responds.

Routines are also roadmaps; they tell us where we're going and how to get there. When we abandon routines, we run the risk of getting lost. But if the potential benefit of doing so is the preservation of our mental faculties, it may be a risk worth taking. In any case, an old saying may come as comfort when we give up routines and risk losing our way: "The only people who get anywhere interesting are the people who get lost."[5]

Abandoning routines and roadmaps and plunging into mystery are certain to lead to mistakes, but making mistakes is a crucial step in learning. Committing errors may also have led to our capacity as a species *to* learn. As Lewis Thomas said, "It was only by making mistakes that mankind blundered toward brains."[6]

The above research findings suggest that we need mystery and that we should cultivate it as a health strategy. In addition to tracking our blood pressure and cholesterol level, we should also be asking, How is this novel going to end? What's forty-nine across? What will my painting or needlepoint look like when it's finished?

If activities such as these are as valuable as the studies suggest, there may be good reasons why elderly widows are chatting around bingo tables in the nation's retirement homes, while their deceased husbands, who weren't much interested in puzzles and games, aren't.

One of those ladies was my widowed mother-in-law, who at eighty-six lived in a retirement village in Little Rock. Six months before her death she volunteered for a study at the local medical school involving a new drug for age-related cognitive decline. She was disqualified when tests showed that her mental capacity was normal: there was nothing the drug could help. This mildly irritated her because she was eager to make a contribution to medical science. She was a poster child for activities that involve mini-mysteries—bridge and other card games, puzzles, and reading, as well as a level of social involvement that fatigued me to think about. Barbara and I dined with her in the retirement center's main building. On entering we passed a reading area and a library with an extraordinary range of books. Then I noticed a table in an alcove on which a large jigsaw puzzle was spread. The several chairs around the table indicated that it was a communal project that brought people together. Then we went to the coatroom, which, I discovered, doubled as the jigsaw puzzle storage area. This was the Fort Knox of jigsaw puzzles, a hundred or more, the largest cache of puzzles I've ever seen. I remarked to my wife, "Someone in the administration has been reading the studies."

Religion and Mystery

Obliterate life's unknowns and it flattens into an insipid sameness. Restore mystery and the pulse quickens; we become livelier and more engaged with the world and the people in it. If we are lucky, mystery may even lead to understanding. As author Lesley Hazelton puts it, "Mystery is wonder, literally, in the sense that we can say, 'I wonder . . .' If we can keep our minds open, rejecting the security of conviction and foregoing certainty for possibility, we then—perhaps—approach what could be called truth."[7]

Yet, for all its truth value, there is an undeclared war on mystery. That is what religious fundamentalism is all about—reducing the mysteries of life into fixed rules and dogmas. But as many wisdom traditions caution, the holy texts on which the dogmas are based are fingers pointing to the moon, not the moon itself. The Absolute is unfathomable and unknowable—alpha *and* omega, the first *and* the last. Dogmas may be comforting, but they are a pale substitute for the real thing, which is always obscured in mystery. Thus the saying: "A religion without its mysteries is a temple without a God."[8]

Some religious folk pull back from "spirituality" these days because it involves, they believe, a freewheeling lack of rigor and discipline and a flirtation with superstition. But the antipathy toward spirituality may reflect, more than anything else, intolerance of mystery. But turning away from religious mystery is dangerous, for without an acceptance of ambiguity we risk becoming slaves to rigid rules that often lead to fanaticism and retribution toward "the other," as we have seen throughout history in religious wars and in the current scourge of religion-based terrorism.

Science and Mystery

Science begins with mystery. Without mystery there would be nothing for scientists *to* discover. In order to do good science, one must first be mystified, baffled, puzzled. As science writer Isaac Asimov explained, "The most exciting phrase to hear in science, the one that heralds new discoveries, is not 'Eureka!' (I found it!) but 'That's funny . . .'"[9]

Sir Francis Bacon (1561–1626), the English philosopher widely regarded as the founder of modern science, marveled at the mystery of the world. "There is no Excellent Beauty," he said, "that hath not some strangeness in the Proportion."[10]

Science also ends in mystery. For all the utopian talk these days of a final theory that will be so simple it can be worn on a T-shirt, it is clear that each discovery opens onto other unknowns—the endlessly receding horizon.

Those who have peered deepest into science know this. Aldous Huxley, who was from one of the great scientific families of England, observed, "We have learnt that nothing is simple and rational except what we ourselves have invented; that God thinks neither in terms of Euclid nor of Riemann; that science has 'explained' nothing; that the more we know the more fantastic the world becomes and the profounder the surrounding darkness. . . ."[11]

Courting Mystery: Wilderness

When we have too little mystery in our lives, a "mystery deficiency syndrome" can develop that is as real as any other physical ailment. One of the best ways of preventing this malady is repeatedly to expose ourselves to wild places.

As a child, I was immersed in nature. Beyond the open fields that surrounded our farmhouse was a forbidding stretch of woods and a labyrinth of creeks and gullies that seemed never to end. I was fascinated by this area and would periodically venture into it—but not too far, because my fascination was always trumped by fear. I had often glimpsed four-footed creatures I could not identify dashing through underbrush, and I'd encountered snakes longer than I was tall. Though terrified, I always returned. One day, in a spasm of bravado, I resolved that I would walk to the other side of the woods without stopping. I never made it. Less than an hour later I was in full retreat. These mysterious woods continued to have their way with me, even after I grew up and left the farm. They still appear in dreams occasionally, down to the minute details of trails and trees and shadows.

I have been spellbound by wild places ever since. I am particularly infatuated by fly-fishing, which often takes place in remote areas. Standing in cold, rushing water, casting tiny bits of feather and fur to trout, one seems to descend—ascend?—to the level of consciousness of the fish themselves. Water is a universal symbol of mystery and the unconscious. Fly-fishing, then, involves standing in mystery, as does any other genuine encounter with wilderness.

Wilderness leads to the sacred, *is* sacred. Willi Unsoeld (1926–1979), the mountaineer and educator who in 1963 was one of the first Americans to climb Mount Everest, describes how as a child he felt his "soul tremble," as if he were "being flooded with a numinous presence," when he had his first wilderness experience.[12] He realized that something momentous had occurred. "For me," he says, "God was no longer to be found in traditional steeple houses, but rather to dwell more vividly among the bare austerities of Earth's high places."

Unsoeld found an explanation of his experience in Rudolf Otto's classic book *The Idea of the Holy*.[13] Otto used the Latin phrase *mysterium tremendum et fascinans*—a tremendous and overpowering mystery—to describe mystical experience. This resonated with Unsoeld. "One can never be completely at ease in the presence of the sacred," he says. "The power is so marked—of such a different dimension—that it comes across as 'wholly other' from our ordinary experiences. The element of mystery is intrinsic to the sacred. It is not a matter merely of not yet knowing all the answers—of simply waiting for further research results to get clear about what we are dealing with. It is rather a basic principle of 'hiddenness'—of sacred realms and dimensions, which must by their very nature remain forever beyond our limited grasp."

The *mysterium tremendum* of wilderness enthralls us—Otto's *fascinans*. "Which is why," says Unsoeld, ". . . people climb mountains—and continue to do so long after they should have 'learned better.' Or run rivers, or sail the seas, or simply go for a walk in the woods. The ripple of the hairs on the back of your neck or the simple eager expectation with which you approach the next wilderness corner testifies to the eagerness with which an encounter with the sacred is sought."

Wisdom traditions the world over tell us that one of the greatest obstacles to the sacred is the ego. Wilderness experience has a way of stopping ego in its tracks. It is simply impossible to maintain an exaggerated sense of self during a prolonged wilderness experience. This is why Unsoeld, after decades of mountaineering, came to regard exposure to wilderness "as a natural path to self-abnegation," in which "the concerns of self evaporate as the flakes of a summer snow flurry before the intense rays of the summer sun."

As the self fades, the sacred can come into clearer view. This is why pre-modern peoples went to wild places on solitary vision quests, hoping to open direct channels to the divine. For generations, millions of Boy and Girl Scouts the world over have been provided a homeopathic taste of this experience, which is surely one of the reasons the scouting movement has endured. A scout is someone who goes ahead, peers into the mysteries, and is sometimes changed by what she has seen, as many young scouts are, even by overnight campouts and summer camp. Today several organizations exist that enable individuals to penetrate more deeply the *mysterium tremendum* that is wilderness, such as Outward Bound, which Unsoeld helped establish, and NOLS, the National Outdoor Leadership School.

Mystery has risks, of course, and the mystery of wilderness can be a siren song luring one beyond a point of no return: *fascinans* with a vengeance. The mystery haters sense this, fear this, and never tire of warning others of the "dreamy mysticism" they believe "nature lovers" are prone to. While admittedly there are a few hermits who never come back after venturing into the wilds, these concerns are overheated. Far more lives have been transformed positively by wilderness mysteries than have been rendered dissolute. As with most things, balance is the key. Unsoeld again: "Why not stay out there in the wilderness the rest of your days . . . ? Because that's not where men are. . . . The final test for me of the legitimacy of the experience is 'How well does your experience of the sacred in nature enable you to cope more effectively with the problems of mankind when you come back to the city?'"[14]

If mystery heals, as evidence suggests, and if wilderness is a source of mystery, we should respect, conserve, and protect it. In the end, we preserve not just wilderness and mystery but our collective sanity as well. As Pulitzer Prize–winning author Wallace Stegner warned, "Something will have gone out of us as a people if we ever let the remaining wilderness be destroyed; if we permit the last virgin forests to be turned into comic books and plastic cigarette cases; if we drive the few remaining members of the wild species into zoos or to extinction; if we pollute the last clean air and dirty the last clean streams and push our paved roads through the last of the silence, so that never again will Americans be free from noise, the exhausts, the stinks of human and automotive waste. And so that never again can we have the chance to see ourselves single, separate, vertical and individual in the world, part of the environment of trees and rocks and soil, brother to the other animals, part of the natural world and competent to belong in it. . . . We simply need that wild country available to us, even if we never do more than drive to its edge and look in. For it can be a means of reassuring ourselves of our sanity as creatures, a part of the geography of hope."[15]

If mystery is healing, what does it heal? One thing is arrogance and hubris. "Mystery" is related to the Greek *myein*, to close the mouth or eyes—to be quiet, to surrender one's self-importance. The natural world is a great teacher of meekness and modesty, as those who spend their lives confronting the *mysterium tremendum* of nature learn. Thus the prayer of Breton fishermen: "O God, thy sea is so great, and my boat is so small," which was engraved on a plaque that President John F. Kennedy, himself a man of the sea, kept on his desk.[16] The same message was expressed more prosaically by rock musician Frank Zappa: "In the fight between you and the world, back the world."[17]

In his essay "Wilderness as Metaphor for Mystery," scientist-engineer-conservationist Rick Van Wagenen describes how modern backpackers into remote areas experience lessons in humility, lessons rooted in prehistory: "Night settles in and the stars come out. A small group of comrades share the meager warmth and light of a dying fire. It has been like this for small bands of travelers and hunters for more than a million years . . . Stories are told of terrible creatures that live in the forest . . . The elders retreat to the warmth of their sleeping bags and the already dreaming children. Outside, noises taunt the dark stillness. . . . Who or what is out there? Better not to know. It is all part of the grand mystery."[18]

One doesn't have to quake at things that go bump in the night to have one's pride punctured by nature. Hubris is generally short-lived in all truly wild places, and those who cannot let go of arrogance often are, too. In my fly-fishing adventures, I have often lost my footing and been dunked in turbulent, frigid trout streams. Each time this happens I wonder if I will survive, and I invariably emerge with a shrunken sense of self-importance—and my experiences are minor compared with those who have survived an avalanche, a storm at sea, or a fall while mountaineering.

Over the years I've come to value the risk that is inherent in wilderness experiences. Risk implies uncertainty and is thus a gateway to mystery. I should not like to fly-fish in a river that could not kill me; the experience would be too predictable, too devoid of mystery and its nourishment of the soul.

Saving Ourselves

Rollo May, one of the most influential psychotherapists of the twentieth century, said, "Now boredom is the loss of the capacity to wonder, to appreciate the sense of mystery and awe in life. Here we are haunted by [astronomer] Harlow Shapley's conclusion as he pondered the possible causes of the destruction of Western Civilization; he cites, along with nuclear war, a radical climate change, a plague, and the simple condition of boredom. Our planet may die because we have become simply bored. It is already observable in some groups as a sense of dullness, joylessness and apathy."[19]

It doesn't have to be this way. Ways of annulling boredom and rekindling a sense of wonder and mystery are limitless. The first step always involves creating a space for mystery to enter—getting quiet in contemplation, meditation, or a walk in the woods. Or we can take up a hobby that silences the mind and introduces uncertainty: painting, making music, baking bread or soufflés, or—my favorite—fly-fishing, which is one of the most advanced forms of uncertainty I know of. We can frequent art museums, attend concerts, or hang out with artists and musicians. We can practice re-thinking the obvious, as artists are always doing. (Picasso's observation, for example: "Computers are worthless. They can only give you answers.") Or we can volunteer in a soup kitchen, grow a garden, or take up stargazing or kite flying. We can expose ourselves to nature—wilderness if possible, or a public park or our backyard, if not. If you're right-handed, do everything with your left hand for twenty-four hours. If you're an intellectual, change your car's sparkplugs yourself; if you're a manual type, read *War and Peace*. The idea is to do something that won't compute and that shatters routines, something that is off the map of personal experience, something strange, uncertain, mysterious.

If May is correct, not only will activities like these relieve boredom and restore mystery, they just might save our skins.

14

Miracles

In order to be a realist you must believe in miracles.

—DAVID BEN-GURION

When a serious illness goes away suddenly, completely, and unexpectedly, we often call it a miracle cure. These events are examples of the extraordinary healing power of ordinary things, because what triggers them is usually commonplace, such as a simple prayer.

During my medical training, I was taught to ignore healings that seemed miraculous. Once, when I asked one of my professors why a lung cancer in a particular patient had disappeared without treatment, he simply shrugged and said, "We see this," and changed the subject. Another professor ascribed this development to "the natural course of the disease." The subtle message seemed to be, some things just happen, things that are so mysterious it's best to ignore them and not ask questions. It's as if the terrain of miracles had a big OFF LIMITS signed posted right in the middle of it.

Yet, how does one ignore someone like Rita Klaus?[1,2] As a twenty-year-old cloistered nun, she developed her first symptoms of multiple sclerosis in 1960. Unable to meet the demands of convent life, she was given dispensation from her vows, finished her college degree in biology, and became a science teacher in a junior high school outside Pittsburgh. She married and had three children. Her disease progressed rapidly and soon she was confined to a wheelchair, with complete paralysis of both feet and ankles. Contractures and muscle spasms caused deformities of her legs, along with intractable sciatic pain. Certain she would never walk again, her doctors surgically severed the tendons in her legs that kept her kneecaps in place. This permitted her to hobble short distances inside her house with full-length leg braces and forearm crutches.

Although formerly extremely religious, her spiritual beliefs evaporated like a snowball on a hot stove. "It's a bunch of malarkey," she said. "God does not intervene in the natural order. Every time I see these televangelist creeps, I feel like puking."

In spite of her rejection of her former beliefs, she allowed her husband to take her to a church service where healing was performed, during which she was prayed over, touched, and hugged. She felt "the strangest experience. . . . There was just this white light, a feeling of absolute love like I'd never felt coursing through me. I felt forgiven and at peace. I wasn't physically healed, but had peace of heart, of knowing I was loved and could weather anything."

The years passed and her disease got worse. Her doctors told her that her nerves and tissue were damaged irreversibly, that there was no hope of improvement, and that it was only a matter of time before she would be bedridden. But in the ensuing years her faith returned and she resumed her prayers. One night she had a dream, which she interpreted as a summons to the healing site in Medjugorje, Yugoslavia. But she had no money to travel—until a month later when someone gave her a financial gift that made the trip possible. On her return home, while she was saying the rosary one day, she heard a gentle voice say, "Why don't you ask?" so she prayed earnestly once again to be healed of MS. She awoke the next day, went to a class in her wheelchair, and began to feel sensations of heat and itching in her lower legs. To her astonishment she realized she could wiggle her toes. Thinking this must be muscle spasms, she dismissed it. Then, when she got home, she bent down to remove her leg braces and noticed that her right kneecap, which had been in a deformed, sideways position since the tendons were cut, had somehow migrated back to its normal position. She said later, "I just remember screaming, 'My God, my God, my leg is straight!'" Then she shed her remaining braces, removed her socks, tucked up her skirt, and said to herself, "If I am cured, I can run up the stairs!"—which she did, all thirteen steps. Her next venture was outdoors. She ran from the house through the woods, jumped a creek, came back covered with leaves and mud, and called her priest, shouting, "I'm healed! I'm healed!" The poor man thought she had gone mad. "I want you to sit down, calm down, take some aspirin, and call your doctor," he stammered. Still babbling, she called a girlfriend, who came over and shared a good cry. The following Monday her husband took her to the rehabilitation hospital. Authors Caryle Hirshberg and Marc Barasch, in their book *Remarkable Recovery*, describe what happened:

> The doctors who convened to examine her were flabbergasted. As the nurses scurried for her charts and patients gawked and craned, the doctors' reactions tellingly varied: [Klaus said,] "One of my doctors saw me and started to laugh. He thought I must have had a twin who I'd brought in to play a practical joke on him." Her neurologist, she says, was "so angry! He said there is no cure for MS, no such thing as miracles. He even called people at the hospital and told them I was a fraud and a fake."[3]

There seemed little doubt about Klaus's cure. Dr. Donald Meisner examined her and found no trace of MS. When word of the case leaked out, he said to a local newspaper, "Spontaneous remissions of multiple sclerosis are possible. The only thing that doesn't fit here is that usually the permanent damage that had occurred up to the point of remission does not go away. In Rita's case, every evidence I could see would suggest that she is totally back to normal."[4]

Some of Klaus's physicians were happy about her recovery. Her urologist, who had last seen her with her bladder swollen to many times normal size and incontinent, retested her and confirmed the organ had returned to normal. "He said there was no way he could explain it, that it was the most beautiful thing he'd ever seen in all his years of practice, and then he cried." Klaus's neurological reports from around that time read,

> Totally independent of any equipment. . . . She has regained full strength of both lower extremities. . . . Her deep tendon reflexes are all symmetrical and normal. . . . A tremendous recovery, I am not sure where to place it in this short period of time. The patient did not get tired of demonstrating to me how good she was . . . I am very happy . . .[5]

Rita Klaus's case is telling. It reveals a spectrum of response from doctors when we are confronted with unexpected, miracle-type cures, ranging from joy and befuddlement to revulsion and horror.

In fact, the idea of miracle cures causes more emotional and intellectual indigestion in my profession than practically any other concept. Some consider miracles an insult to science because these events presumably violate the laws of nature—although it is more likely our understanding of physical laws, not the laws themselves, that is violated. Other physicians harbor the belief that victory over a disease like far-advanced MS ought to be hard-fought and hard-won; Rita Klaus's case, in which advanced MS simply goes away, makes a mockery of the heroic efforts of medical science and should be set aside.

Indeed, cases such as Klaus's make conventional medicine seem clumsy and inadequate. This is not a happy thought for some doctors. One woman, who suffered from severe macular degeneration and partial blindness, reported to me her experience with her ophthalmologist

when her disease went away following prayers by a healer. After examining her eyes and confirming her recovery, the physician flew into a
rage. He screamed at her that miracle cures don't happen, and he told
her to leave his office, find another doctor, and never come back.

You'd think we physicians would be eager to report miracle cures
in scientific journals as an opportunity for deeper understanding, but
we are not. Take the case of four-year-old Ann O'Neill, who was hospitalized with acute lymphocytic leukemia during Easter week in Baltimore in 1952.[6] At the time, this disease was 100 percent fatal. The
priest had given her the final rites, and her aunt had already prepared
her burial garment, a hand-stitched gown of lovely yellow silk. When
the head pediatrics nurse asked the little girl if she'd like to go to
heaven, Ann's feisty mother said, "No, Sister, not yet." Dr. John
Healy, a pediatrics resident at the time, has vivid recollections of the
all-consuming faith of Ann's mother. "She never even questioned for
five seconds that this girl was going to get better," he recalls. Shortly
thereafter, Ann's parents bundled her up, took her out of the hospital
into the rain, to the cemetery where Mother Elizabeth Seton, a
revered Catholic nun, lay buried. There, surrounded by praying nuns,
they laid her on the tomb and asked for a healing.

Back in the hospital, blood tests a few days later showed no trace
of cancer. Ann's physicians were baffled. When word of the apparent
miracle reached Rome, Vatican investigators trooped to Baltimore to
see for themselves. Nine years later, the Church insisted that Ann
undergo a bone marrow biopsy to confirm her cure. At this stage,
Dr. Sidney Farber, the well-known Harvard pathologist who had pioneered the first effective treatment for leukemia, oversaw the investigation. Dr. Milton Sacks, Ann's physician and one of the country's
foremost hematologists, testified at the Vatican tribunal that she
should not have survived in view of her 105-degree fever, severe ane-
mia, and the bloody sores on her neck and back. He emphasized that,
at the time, her disease was "inexorably fatal." Eventually the Pope
declared Ann a miracle, and not long afterward canonized Mother
Seton an American saint.[7]

Oddly, this sensational case was never reported in the medical literature. Hematologist Dr. Milton Sacks told a *Washington Post* reporter in 1993, "The only reason this case has not been written up is that I have been afraid to."[8] This is one reason miracle-type cures are not considered more frequent.

It is common practice in medical journals actually to disguise miracle-type responses. Consider, for example, how survival statistics are analyzed. In one study of survivors of untreated breast cancer, the median survival time (the point at which half the patients had died) was 3.3 years. But this figure, mentioned only in passing in the report, was obtained by omitting two cases in which the women survived for 40 years following their diagnosis without treatment.[9] These cases, called "outliers," are routinely omitted because they lie far outside the statistical norm. Most people would probably think that researchers should focus on these cases, because they might contain clues for survival that could be extended to all women with breast cancer. But no; paradoxically, the researchers highlight those patients who die early rather than those who live long. In my opinion, ignoring these extraordinary cases borders on intellectual dishonesty.

The Patient Gets Left Out

When unexpected cures are reported in professional journals, they are invariably drained of every drop of emotional, psychological, and spiritual juice the experiences may have held for the patient. Physicians who report these cases usually mention physical factors that might have played a role in triggering the response, such as infection, which is known sometimes to boost the immune system's resistance to cancer, but almost never are psychological factors acknowledged as playing a possible role. Why the blackout on the psyche? As psychologists G. B. Challis and H. J. Stam, of the University of Calgary, report in their investigation of cases of spontaneous regression of cancer, "No physician was willing to risk his/her reputation by reporting a case of spontaneous regression he/she felt was due to a psychological method."[10]

It is as if the patient has no mind, emotions, spirit, or soul, but is only a mass of molecules and meat. Consider a case that was written up in 1990 in *Gut*.[11] It involves Muriel Bourne-Mullen, a seventy-one-year-old British geriatric nurse. She grew up in India during the 1920s and 1930s, the daughter of the British Army officer who arrested Mahatma Gandhi. She was nourished on the spiritual lore of Hinduism and often witnessed religious ceremonies. Although a devout Catholic all her life and devoted to daily prayer, she honored all faiths. In 1987 she discovered she had liver cancer that had metastasized to her lungs. Her doctors gave her six months to live, and told her that her condition was so far advanced that treatment would be "quite unnecessary."

Although Bourne-Mullen had a place in her belief system for the mysterious and the inexplicable, she considered herself a critical thinker. Her childhood in India had exposed her to methods of healing unknown to Western science, but which she could not ignore. In addition, her subsequent experience as a cancer ward nurse prepared her for the unexpected and the unpredictable. Following her diagnosis, she began to pray more diligently and passionately, beseeching St. Jude, patron of lost causes. Her family rallied around her, and others began to pray. In a few months she began gaining weight. Her tumor shrank and then disappeared, confirmed by scans, X-rays, and biopsies. In spite of this, her physician pressured her to undergo a liver transplant, which she refused. She says, "I was perfectly hale and hearty, love. I told him there was not nothing the matter with me and that would be quite unnecessary."[12]

When the case was reported in *Gut*, Bourne-Mullen was fleetingly described as "a sixty-three-year-old white woman with a four-month history of abdominal discomfort and bloating after eating." Then she disappears, replaced by pleomorphic tumor cells with bizarre giant nuclei.

The report confirms the original diagnosis of metastatic liver cancer and that she was discharged home with no treatment, since no therapy was considered worthwhile. Only two published reports in medical history of regression of primary liver tumors exist, the article states, and only one, from China, concerns *metastatic* liver cancer. A litany of possible factors are listed that may have been involved in the regression, such as endocrine and immunologic mechanisms or interruption of the tumor's blood supply. But in the end the physicians throw up their hands and simply acknowledge, with admirable honesty, "The patient received no treatment for the tumour, and regression therefore can be truly described as spontaneous." What is *not* admirable, in my judgment, is the information blackout of Bourne-Mullen—what *she* thought was responsible for a cure, including her spiritual experiences, beliefs, and prayers.

Another Side

The embargo on miracle-type cures mainly concerns academic physicians working in medical schools and teaching hospitals, scholars who have learned to be properly horrified by these events. Doctors in private practice are much more open to these happenings. Most of them see cases of spontaneous remissions from time to time, and in the right circumstances are willing to discuss them.

For several years I have been invited to speak to a national meeting of hundreds of physicians who gather to update their knowledge in the field of internal medicine (Update and Review of Internal Medicine, sponsored by Harvard Medical School, Beth Israel Deaconess Medical Center, and University of New Mexico Sciences Center). My task is to discuss the evidence for the role of spiritual practices and intercessory prayer in health. When I was first invited to give this address, I accepted hesitantly; I doubted that these physicians, who came to refine their conventional knowledge, would have much patience with a lecture on this subject. But after my talk I was amazed at what happened. There was intense interest and discussion, all of which was cordial. These practicing physicians were not only fascinated by the evidence underlying spirituality and prayer as factors in healing, they wanted to tell about miracle-type responses in their own patients. One said, "If you think those cases *you* described were weird, let me tell you about a patient of *mine.*" Several of the doctors met with me afterward to swap stories.

These physicians aren't unique. Sir William Osler (1849–1919), regarded as the father of Western scientific medicine, spoke about the widespread occurrence of miracle-type healings. He said, "Literature is full of examples of remarkable cures through the influence of the imagination, which is only an active phase of faith. . . . Phenomenal, even what could be called miraculous cures, are not very uncommon. Like others, I have had cases any one of which, under suitable conditions, could have been worthy of a shrine or made the germ of a pilgrimage."[13]

A Further Look

Let's look at two cures related to Lourdes, France, the most famous pilgrimage site for healing in the Western world.

In 1962, Vittorio Michelli, a middle-aged Italian man, was admitted to the Military Hospital of Verona, Italy, suffering from a large, excruciatingly painful mass in the left buttock, which was so extensive it limited the range of motion of the hip. X rays revealed extensive destruction of the bones of the pelvis and hip joint. A biopsy, taken in May, showed a fusiform cell carcinoma. Beyond hope of surgery, he was immobilized in a plaster cast and was sent to a regional center for radiotherapy. Four days later, however, he was discharged without receiving any irradiation and was admitted to the Military Hospital at Trente. He spent the next ten months there without any treatment, in spite of ongoing destruction of bone from the tumor, as well as progressive loss of all active movement of the left lower limb and progressive physical deterioration. By this time, Michelli was literally falling apart—the mass continuing to enlarge, eating away the bone and supporting structures that kept his left leg attached to the rest of his body.

On 24 May, 1963, approximately a year after his original diagnosis, emaciated and unable to eat, he was taken by friends to Lourdes. It must have been a difficult journey for Michelli in his plaster cast. On arrival, his friends bathed him in the holy waters. Following his bath, he reported sensations of heat moving through his body, as well as an immediate return of his appetite and a resurgence of energy.

Then his friends lugged him back to the hospital in Trente, still in plaster, where he began to gain weight and become much more active. A month later, his doctors consented to remove his cast and take another X ray and found that the tumor was smaller than before. It continued to diminish, then it disappeared. Continued X rays tracked an astonishing event—the destroyed bone began to regrow and completely reconstructed itself. Two months after his trip to Lourdes, Vittorio Michelli went for a walk. This is what his doctors said:

> A remarkable reconstruction of the iliac bone and cavity has taken place. The X rays made in 1964–5, –8 and –9 confirm categorically and without doubt that an unforeseen and even overwhelming bone reconstruction has taken place of a type unknown in the annals of world medicine. We ourselves, during a university and hospital career of over 45 years spent largely in the study of tumors and neoplasms of all kinds of bone structures and having ourselves treated hundreds of such cases, have never encountered a single spontaneous bone reconstruction of such a nature.
>
> ... [A] medical explanation of the cure ... was sought and none could be found. He did not undergo specific treatment, did not suffer from any susceptible intercurrent infection that might have had any influence on the evolution of the cancer.
>
> A completely destroyed articulation was completely reconstructed without any surgical intervention. The lower limb which was useless became sound, the prognosis is indisputable, the patient is alive and in a flourishing state of health nine years after his return from Lourdes.

This case was declared a miracle by the International Medical Commission of Lourdes (CMIL) in 1970 and was officially recognized by the Catholic Church as a miracle in 1976.[14] The Commission is made up of about two dozen members from Western Europe and England, representing a wide range of specialties including general medicine and surgery, orthopedics, psychiatry, radiology, dermatology, ophthalmology, pediatrics, cardiology, oncology, and neurology. Nearly half the members hold chairs in medical schools. The Commission meets in Paris annually to review cases. At every stage, rigorous attention is given to the thoroughness of documentation including laboratory and biopsy findings. No identifiable physical intervention must be present that might have caused the favorable response, otherwise the case is discarded. The suddenness and completeness of the response is also considered crucial, as well as length of follow-up. The final question is, does the cure of this person constitute a phenomenon which is contrary to the observations and expectations of medical knowledge and is it scientifically inexplicable?

Being declared a miracle cure isn't easy. In 1735, Cardinal Lambertini, who later became Pope Benedict XIV, laid down five rules that have continued to serve as criteria:

1. The disease must be serious, incurable, or unlikely to respond to treatment.
2. The disease which disappeared must not have reached a stage at which it would have resolved by itself.
3. No medication should have been given, or if some medicines were prescribed then they must have had only minimal effects. (Today, it is most unusual to find a case completely untreated; therefore this rule is currently interpreted as excluding any patient who has had a potentially curative treatment unless that treatment can be demonstrated to have failed.)
4. The cure must be sudden and reached instantaneously. (This criterion is now extended to include cures developing over a period of days.)
5. The cure must be complete, not partial or incomplete.[15]

Consider another case passed by the International Medical Commission of Lourdes in 1982, that of Delizia Cirolli, a child from a village on the slopes of Mt. Etna in Sicily. When she was twelve years old she went to a physician with a swollen knee. When an X ray showed bone change, she was referred to the Orthopedic Clinic of the University of Catania. Eventually, a biopsy was interpreted as a bony metastasis from neuroblastoma. When the surgeon recommended amputation, the family refused. He then advised irradiation, but this upset Delizia so greatly that her parents took her home without any treatment. Further consultation was obtained at the University of Turin, but no treatment was given.

Eventually, Delizia's teacher suggested that the family take her to Lourdes, and the locals took up a collection to help finance the trip. In August 1976, Delizia and her mother arrived at Lourdes and spent four days attending ceremonies, praying at the Grotto, and bathing in the water. But there was no obvious improvement in the girl's condition, and X rays the following month showed continued extension of the tumor. Delizia went downhill quickly and the family began to plan for her funeral. In spite of this, the villagers continued to pray fervently to Our Lady of Lourdes for her cure, and her mother continued to administer water from Lourdes.

Shortly before Christmas, Delizia announced she wanted to get up from bed and go outside, which she did without pain, but was unable to venture far because of profound weakness. At this time she weighed only forty-eight pounds but her knee swelling had disappeared, and her general condition normalized.

The following July, she returned to Lourdes and presented herself to the Medical Bureau. Follow-up studies revealed no further evidence of tumor. The exact diagnosis proved difficult, however. The original biopsy slides were presented to eminent French histologists; opinion was split between an undifferentiated neuroblastoma and Ewing's tumor. In either case, her response was remarkable. At the time of her evaluation, "spontaneous remission of neuroblastoma [had] been reported, but very rarely and never after the age of 5 years ... [and] spontaneous remission of Ewing's tumor [had] not been recorded."[16]

How Common?

As of 1984, it was estimated that over two million sick pilgrims had visited Lourdes since 1858.[17] Of these, about 6,000 individuals— 0.3 percent—claimed to be cured and were examined by the doctors who work at Lourdes. Following rigorous evaluation, almost all claims were rejected; only sixty-four (0.003 percent of the total number of sick pilgrims) were eventually recognized as miracle cures by the Catholic Church.[18]

This may seem like a meager harvest, yet it may be that we are looking for miracles in the wrong places. Rather than focusing on high-profile sites such as Lourdes and Medjugorje, perhaps we should be examining peoples' everyday lives. In 2000, a *Newsweek* poll did just that, and found that 63 percent of Americans say they know someone who has experienced a miracle, and 48 percent say they have experienced or witnessed one.[19]

Practicing physicians are not far behind—or perhaps are actually out front—in these beliefs. According to a 1996 poll of American family physicians, 99 percent were convinced that spiritual beliefs can heal, 75 percent said that prayers of others can help a patient recover, and 38 percent believed that faith healers can make people well.[20]

John L. Pfenninger, MD, of Midland, Mich., is one such physician. He is the author of a highly acclaimed medical text for primary-care physicians and a national leader in the field of family practice.[21] I came across his experience with miracle-type healings while researching the role of prayer in healing. At eighteen, his son Matthew developed a rapidly growing, malignant brain tumor. When the cancer defied conventional treatment at Columbia, Pfenninger invited his colleagues to participate in a "Gathering to Heal" ceremony back home at MidMichigan Medical Center in Midland. "What amazed me," he says, "is that 60 out of 110 doctors came. These were the most scientific people imaginable." Ten days later, Matthew's brain tumor had vanished. The specialists taking care of Matthew had no explanation. Matthew endured a stormy course over the next several years with a recurrence. Eventually a bone marrow transplant proved successful. Seven years later, he is a straight-A student in college. Dr. Pfenninger is baffled but comfortable with the mystery of what happened. "We don't know how the power of mind or prayer works," he says, "but that doesn't mean it doesn't work."[22]

I agree. Sometimes in medicine we simply must be tolerant of a bit of mystery. Doing so is simply part of being a good doctor. Throughout the history of medicine, we have often known *that* something works before we understand *how* it works. Examples are legion—aspirin, quinine, citrus for scurvy, penicillin, general anesthetics—and, we can add, miracle-type responses such as Pfenninger's son Matthew.

Miracles and the Mind

Does one's state of mind play a role in miracle cures? Is there a miracle-prone personality?

In many of these cases, the sick individual appears to have important work left undone, and needs to be healed in order to accomplish it. This may kindle a profound desire for healing and may, in unknown ways, set the stage for a dramatic turnaround.

A famous example of the "unfinished business" pattern took place in Europe in the thirteenth century when a zealous young priest developed a painful, grotesque area on his foot, believed to be cancer. He endured his problem without complaining. The lesion worsened, and it was decided that the foot required amputation. He spent the night prior to surgery praying before his crucifix, and sank into light sleep. When he awoke he was totally cured. His doctors, unable to find any evidence of disease, canceled the operation. The young priest believed he had great work ahead of him and needed the time to do it. He dedicated the rest of his life to ministering to patients with cancer, and lived to be eighty. He was later canonized as St. Peregrinus, who is considered the patron saint of the spontaneous regression of cancer.[23]

The "unfinished business" theme appears also in the case of Sister Gertrude of the Sisters of Charity in New Orleans, who was admitted to the Hotel-Dieu Hospital in New Orleans on December 17, 1934. For some months she had been sick, and on admission was suffering from jaundice, severe abdominal pain, nausea, chills, and fever. She was admitted to the care of Dr. James T. Nix, who previously had operated on her for the removal of her gall bladder. Following a provisional diagnosis of cancer of the pancreas, an exploratory laparotomy was performed on January 5, 1935. An inoperable carcinoma of the head of the pancreas was discovered and was confirmed with biopsy by three pathologists.

Sister Gertrude's fellow sisters interceded through prayer with Mother Seton, the deceased founder of the order. Their sick colleague had more work to do, they said, and her life needed to be spared so she could remain in service. She began to improve rapidly and was discharged on February 1, 1934, returning to her duties a month later. Her arduous work continued for seven and a half years. When she died suddenly on August 20, 1942, an autopsy revealed death due to pulmonary embolism, with no evidence of carcinoma of the pancreas.[24]

Support for a miracle-prone state of mind comes from the little town of Medjugorje, in the former Yugoslavia.

On June 24, 1981, an apparition of the Virgin Mary appeared to a group of children in the town. Thereafter, reports of miracle cures began to surface and Medjugorje quickly gained a reputation as "Lourdes East." The late Brendan O'Regan, vice-president for research at the Institute of Noetic Sciences in Sausalito, California, traveled to Medjugorje to investigate these strange happenings.[25] He interviewed Father Slavko, the local priest, who is a Franciscan monk with a PhD in psychology. The priest revealed to O'Regan that he could sometimes tell who would be healed. "It's very often the people who come and don't determinedly *want* healing who are affected," he said. "They come with an open mind and ask for healing but they have not come with this as the single-minded purpose of their trip." O'Regan observed:

> This [suggests] an interesting psychological profile of those that would be healed and indeed, being in Medjugorje presents one with an intense experiential sense of the presence of simple faith and devotion. Interestingly, one gets the impression that one can easily tell the difference between the devout and the merely pious there. There is a sad, faraway look in the eyes of the devout that is unmistakable. It seems like a kind of yearning for something, the search for a memory, the need for an all-embracing experience of love of a kind not yet found. This alone suggests to the eye seeking clues that these people *are* in a very different place psychologically, emotionally and indeed psychophysiologically.[26]

However, these findings are tentative. On balance, no psychological profile has yet been developed that fully accounts for spontaneous healings. These cures happen not just to those who have saintly dispositions, fierce determination, or positive thoughts, but to reprobates and passive quitters as well. Exceptions can be found to any psychological pattern yet advanced. I rather like this confused state of affairs. It suggests that no one has a monopoly on miracle cures; they are available to anyone, no matter how devout or unsaintly they may be.[27]

Volumes have been written about why some people experience cures from serious illness and others don't. Some say the person who doesn't recover was "too attached" to his or her illness and could not "let go" and "accept healing." Others claim that the individual was too attached to getting well; they desired healing too much. Some say the sick person didn't "love enough" or wasn't "forgiving enough," which doomed his or her chances for recovery. These explanations have always seemed like desperate floundering to me. Although they may seem applicable in isolated cases, they make sweeping generalizations and are hopelessly incomplete. They trivialize illness and the complex interactions of mind and body, and, worst of all, they often blame the victim for not getting well. We ought to come clean and admit the obvious: in most cases *we don't know* why spontaneous healings happen.

Why Is the Debate About Miracles So Vehement?

There is a strange coterie of humans who devote their lives to attacking what they consider the irrational beliefs of others, often with great fanfare. Although they refer to themselves as skeptics, this term is misleading and far too flattering. "Skeptic" is from the Greek *skeptikos*, meaning "thoughtful, inquiring." A genuine skeptic, according to Webster's, is "a person who habitually doubts, questions, or suspends judgment upon matters generally accepted."[28] Skepticism is a valuable and honored tradition within science, and science cannot thrive without it. However, individuals who loathe miracles and assault those who believe in them are untrue to authentic skepticism, because they do not suspend judgment; their minds are already made up.

As a result of my writings about the scientific evidence for prayer, I was once invited to be a guest on a television program about miracles. Also present were two women, both quite religious, who believed they had experienced a miracle. One had seen an apparition of the Virgin Mary, which had been witnessed by hundreds of other individuals. The other woman claimed that her rosary beads had turned to gold as she prayed to Jesus. A theologian was present to represent the Church's views on such matters. The most animated guest was a professional debunker who had written a book about the folly of miracles. After the women described their experiences, he attacked them with a vengeance. He gleefully shredded their stories, offered physical explanations for what they experienced, and essentially condemned them as fools. The joy and sense of wonder drained from these simple, devout women. Both began to weep, trying to blot their tears without being noticed by the television cameras. When the debunker was finished, he sat back in obvious satisfaction, having once again manned the barricades of reason against miracle-loving barbarians.

Why such vehemence?

Hard-core materialists believe the idea of a miracle is absurd. They are convinced that the so-called ironclad laws of nature, which cannot be breached, dictate all events in nature. Because miracles require a temporary suspension of natural law, miracles cannot exist, by definition. Other individuals, however, often including highly credentialed scientists, believe that the laws of nature are not absolute; they can be suspended temporarily, permitting miracles to happen. And in any case, they say, because our knowledge of nature's laws is incomplete, we should be cautious in declaring what can and cannot happen.

Since the dawn of science, the arguments on both sides have often been vitriolic, with theologians using miracles as evidence for the Divine, and rationalists condemning them in defense of reason. Following the Enlightenment, it was a badge of intellectual courage to dismiss miracles and to consider those who believed in them as traitors to reason. "Crush the infamy," Voltaire railed in eighteenth-century France, referring to claims of miraculous healings.[29] Even Thomas Jefferson appeared embarrassed by miracles. "[He] was as dictatorial as the Grand Inquisitor when he published a version of the Bible bowdlerizing all references to miracles!" notes philosopher Michael Grosso.[30] Freud also took up the antimiracle drumbeat and wove it into his psychology in works such as *The Future of an Illusion*.[31] For Freud, Grosso says, miracles were so much "spiritual tinsel . . . [and] religion is a feint, a teddy bear for neurotics, an anti-reality racket—in short, an illusion."[32]

One reason the debate about miracles is so mean-spirited is due to our tenacious defense of our worldview. Our worldview—the assumptions, usually unconscious, about how and why the universe behaves as it does—influences how we see ourselves in relation to the physical world. In some deep sense, we *are* our worldview. If I question your worldview, I'm suggesting that you don't know how the world behaves, and that you are out of touch with reality. Since being out of touch with reality is a characteristic of psychosis, I am accusing you of being insane. Debates about miracles, which are really debates about worldviews, therefore involve veiled charges of madness. It is no wonder they are so bitter.

Some people's worldview is so precious to them that they would rather forego a miracle than modify it. Writer Joseph Cary is admirably honest on this score. "I dimly see that I want to be helped," he says, "but on my own terms only: I don't believe in miracles for me."[33]

But it isn't just scientists who oppose miracles; theologians get skittish about them too. Miracles confront theologians with a blizzard of pesky questions. Why does God confer miracles on only a few? Is God unfair and capricious? Why would the Almighty construct a world in which miracles were needed in the first place, i.e., why do disease and suffering exist? If the Divine constructed the natural laws, why would s/he then violate them by allowing miracles?

I believe miracles represent not chaos, but the insertion of order into the disordered processes of disease. Neuro-ophthalmologist Christian Wertenbaker expresses this point of view: "[A] characteristic of miracles is that they involve the unlikely creation of order. Restoration of life to a dead person, or of health or sight to a sick one, . . . are all examples."[34]

Those who protest miracles are like a man dying of thirst who complains about the temperature of the water he's offered. You'd think we'd be more grateful. In any case, all the scientific, philosophical, and theological arguments that have been offered throughout history in opposition of miracles do not erase the experiences of a Rita Klaus, a Vittorio Michelli, a Delizia Cirolli, a Muriel Bourne-Mullen, or an Ann O'Neill. These dazzling events fortunately do not cease to exist merely because we disapprove of them.

False Hope and Other Cautions

Many spiritual traditions have warned against getting caught up in the miraculous. When we do, we can be diverted from more important spiritual objectives. An example of this universal caution comes from the Persian mystic Ansâri:

> *If thou canst walk on water*
> *Thou art no better than a straw.*
> *If thou canst fly in the air*
> *Thou art no better than a fly.*
> *Conquer thy heart*
> *That thou mayest become somebody.*[35]

Others warn that miracles may lead to unintended consequences. As Patrick Harper, the inimitable army sergeant in Bernard Cornwell's Sharpe novels, says, "You don't want a miracle. They always turn out bad. . . . St. Patrick turns out all the snakes from Ireland and what happens? We get so bored that we let the English in to take their place. The poor man must be turning in his grave. Snakes were better."[36]

A widespread concern is that talk of miracles creates false hope. Of course, it is possible to create false hope by focusing exclusively on the miraculous, but the same charge can be made against any other therapy. Any intervention can be oversold, such as penicillin, which is worthless in many of the bacterial infections for which it was once considered a miracle drug. Or consider exercise, which can have serious and even lethal side effects. Should we stop recommending exercise because some people develop sore knees or drop dead while jogging?

Others say miracle talk leads to guilt. If people pray for a miracle cure and nothing happens, they will conclude that they are unworthy. Thus many health-care professionals conclude that the risk of false hope and guilt are so great that the miracle dialogue should be shut down altogether. I suggest that those individuals who simply cannot imagine how hope can be extended to the sick without risking false expectations or guilt consider another line of work—perhaps repairing not humans but automobiles or computers, where hope and positive thinking aren't as important. Spontaneous miracle-type cures are a blessed fact of history. It would be unethical and cruel to deliberately hide them from anyone who is desperately ill, for whom hope in any form would be a comfort.

Miracles: Beyond Curing

Miracles are about far more than curing disease.

"Miracle" is derived from the Latin verb *mirari*, to wonder or marvel. The suffix *-cle* turns it into a noun: a miracle is that which provokes awe or wonder.

Why is it important to wonder about things? Wonder, said Aristotle, is the beginning of wisdom—and miracles, by stimulating wonder, can set the stage for becoming wiser.

Michael Grosso, one of our wisest observers of miracles, emphasizes this point. "Our worldviews have become so hardened," he says, "so sealed to the mystery of being, that we need to be confounded by miracles. It almost seems as if some impish Mind Out There likes to shock and surprise us, as if it wants to disarm our arrogant intellects. [They] keep our conceptual grids loose and flexible. They prevent hardening of our conceptual arteries. They inspire wonder and keep the soul young."[37]

Critics often charge that those who believe in miracles are so unhappy with their ordinary lives that they are easily overcome by illusions, fantasies, and vague religious impulses. But why is it a bad thing to wonder about "something more," or to sense that a numinous, transcendent quality of the universe might manifest in one's life, perhaps miraculously? Grosso continues,

> Many hold that our view of the world has been stripped bare, made one-dimensional by mechanistic reductionists, had its

depth, color, and soul eviscerated. The [domain of miracles] has something to offer this depressed ontology. The spiritual imagination lights up with a fresh metaphysical glow, once we concede that a miraculous . . . factor is at large. Given this factor, a new spirit of optimism becomes possible; for example, we are entitled to believe that miraculous healings are part of the possible nature we inhabit.[38]

And what is this "possible nature"? Grosso again:

It is as if miracles—their apparent impetus to transcend death, time, space, and matter—want to create a new environment, a new niche of being for the next stage of our evolutionary adventure. And what is that adventure? To advance toward increasing likeness to God. Put together a composite image of where all the extraordinary powers and miracle data seem to be pointing, and a new model of the human emerges, an opening to a new environment. Miracles are not about titillating hyperphysical acrobatics; their importance lies in the fact that *they foreshadow a revolution in our understanding the structure of human reality itself.*[39]

What Do Patients Believe?

I have known many individuals who experienced miracle cures, and all of them were humbled by the experience. Like Grosso, they sensed that the significance of their healing went beyond the disappearance of their disease and pointed to the divine. This conviction can be so profound that they are reluctant to talk about their healing, as if the proper response is silence and gratitude, not words. Nonetheless these individuals invariably have ideas about why the miracle occurred. Almost always their reasons are commonplace, which is why miracle cures belong in our tally of extraordinary healing events that are triggered by ordinary things.

One reason why the recipients of miracles are reluctant to talk about them is the sheer ordinariness of these triggering events. One woman I know says that no one would believe her if she stated publicly that she sang her tumor away. Another highly educated woman who was scheduled for surgery for cervical cancer prayed for healing, then "got hot all over." When the surgeon repeated her examination just prior to surgery, the cancer had vanished and the operation was canceled. She refused to tell her story on a national television program exploring miracle cures because she felt it was "not fancy enough" and no one would believe her. A man whose cancer went away after he embarked on a strenuous exercise program said his healing was "nobody else's business." These responses are so consistent that I have come to regard humility as a key aspect of the miracle story.

We *All* Believe in Miracles

An unanswered question in science, which occurs to every wide-eyed child, is, why does anything exist? Why is there something rather than nothing? Scientists come closest to these queries when they ask what existed before the Big Bang, the primordial explosion that signaled the beginning of the universe. The answer generally given is, "Nothing." By any stretch of the imagination, this is the greatest miracle ever conceived. If scientists are willing to believe that something as stupendous as the entire universe came from nothing, it's difficult to imagine what they would *not* believe. If skeptics can swallow the tenets of modern cosmology about the origins of the Universe, why should they go ballistic when a simple cancer up and disappears when splashed with a little holy water?

Modern scientists are swimming in a veritable soup of miracles, which most of them don't realize. Scientists have their gods—matter, energy, space-time—and they ascribe to them qualities that are as miraculous as anything that religionists impute to the Divine. For example, scientists speak of the *eternality* and *immutability* of natural laws, the *indestructibility* of matter and energy, and the space-time invariance or *omnipresence* of the physical laws. In a religious context, these would be considered attributes of the Absolute.

Sometimes a scientist—often a very great scientist—realizes that miracles pervade everything. Einstein was such a person. As he put it, "There are only two ways to live your life: one is as though nothing is a miracle, the other is as though everything is a miracle."[40]

We are on the verge of a transformation of the debate about the miraculous. Today, science is teeming with new ideas about the nature of consciousness and its role in the world. As these views become more widely known, miracle cures will cease to seem less blasphemous scientifically, and more scientists will feel free to investigate them.

In the meantime, those who believe in the possibility of spontaneous cures should be patient. It hardly matters that current scientific theories do not embrace miracles. Miracles will endure; most current theories won't. And to those religious folk who fear that science will debase miracles if one day it can explain them, fret not. Science cannot sanitize miracles. It is, rather, the other way around: The study of miracles can transform and enrich science.

When Wilbur and Orville Wright invented the airplane, the experts considered human flight impossible. In spite of this, the Wright brothers learned the principles of flight, how to turn and steer their plane, and how to manufacture one. Although they flew their plane up and down and around over two main highways and a railroad track for five years, the experts took little notice.[41] Even though commuters could look out the windows of their trains and see them doing so, the newspapers they were reading at that very moment decreed that it was completely impossible for a machine heavier than air to fly.[42]

We are in a similar situation with miracle cures. While experts assure us that they are impossible, they keep on happening. If we look out the windows of everyday experience, we can see them for ourselves.

When we are confronted with a spectacular cure that lies outside our current understanding, we need not agonize about whether or not it was *really* a miracle. We can be grateful that it happened, and we can strive for greater understanding of what occurred. If we are lucky, we may find out. If not, we can be thankful that the universe behaves in benevolent ways.

By any measure, a miracle.

Notes

Introduction

1. Starfield, B. Is U.S. health really the best in the world? *Journal of the American Medical Association.* 2000; 284(4): 483–485.

2. *Webster's New World Dictionary.* 2nd college ed., s.v. "ordinary." (New York: Prentice Hall, 1986), 1001.

3. Ibid., s.v. "plain."

4. Ibid., s.v. "simple."

5. *Bartlett's Familiar Quotations,* 16th ed., s.v. "Stendhal." (Boston: Little, Brown, 1992), 396.

6. www.wisdomquotes.com/cat_simplicity.html (accessed January 29, 2005).

7. *Bartlett's Familiar Quotations,* 16th ed., s.v. "Tolstoi."

8. van der Rohe quoted on www.greatbuildings.com/architects/Ludwig_Mies_van_der_Rohe.html (accessed January 31, 2005).

9. Venturi quoted on www.josephsoninstitute.org/quotes/quotesimplicity.htm (accessed January 29, 2005).

1. Optimism

1. Halifax-Grof, J. "Hex death," in *Parapsychology and Anthropology: Proceedings of an International Conference Held in London, August 29–31, 1973.* Allan Angoff and Diana Barth, eds. (New York: Parapsychology Foundation, 1974), 59–79.

2. Klopfer, B. Psychological variables in human cancer. *Journal of Projective Techniques.* 1957; 21: 331–340.

3. Weil, A. *Spontaneous Healing* (New York: Alfred A. Knopf, 1995), 63–64.

4. Lown, B. *The Lost Art of Healing* (New York: Houghton-Mifflin, 1996), 65.

5. Weil, A. op. cit., 61.

6. Seligman, M.E.P. *Learned Optimism* (New York: Alfred A. Knopf, 1991), 111.

7. The science of happiness: why optimists live longer. *Time,* January 17, 2005. Front cover.

8. Stendahl quoted on www.josephsoninstitute.org/quotes/quotehappiness. htm (accessed January 29, 2005).

9. Eckhart, M. *Sermons and Collations,* XCIX, in *A Dazzling Darkness: An Anthology of Western Mysticism,* ed. Grant, Patrick (Grand Rapids, Mich.: William B. Eerdmans, 1985), 343.

10. *Bartlett's Familiar Quotations,* 16th ed., s.v. "Julian of Norwich."

11. Angelou, M., quoted on www.quotemore.com/dp/2-8.htm (accessed January 17, 2005).

12. Dossey, L. *Recovering the Soul* (New York: Bantam, 1989), 1–11.

13. Jamison, K.R. *An Unquiet Mind* (New York: Alfred A. Knopf, 1995).

14. Jamison, K.R. *Exuberance: The Passion for Life* (New York: Alfred A. Knopf, 2004).

15. Hubbard, E., in Auden, W.H., and Kronenberger L., eds. *The Viking Book of Aphorisms* (New York: Barnes & Noble, 1993), 56.

16. Else, L. The passionate life. *New Scientist.* November 2004; 184(2475): 44–47. Interview of Jamison, K.R.

17. The tsunami was a punishment from Allah for celebrating Christmas and other sins. See http://www.Schwartzreport.net, 11 January, 2004 (accessed January 12, 2004). Many similar comments were recorded and translated by the MEMRI TV Monitor Project. See MEMRI TV Monitor Project, www.memri.org/bin/latestnews.cgi?ID=SD84205.

18. Miller, H., in Sunbeams. *The Sun,* April 1999; 280: 48.

19. *Bartlett's Familiar Quotations,* 16th ed., s.v. "Montesquieu."

20. Justice, B. *Who Gets Sick: How Beliefs, Moods, and Thoughts Affect Your Health* (Houston: Peak Press, 2000), 63.

21. Ibid., 64.

22. Hinkle, L.E., Wolff, H.G. Health and the social environment: Experimental investigations, in Leighton, A.H., Clausen, J.A., and Wilson, R.N., eds. *Explorations in Social Psychiatry* (New York: Basic Books, 1957) 105–132. See also Hinkle, L.E., Christenson, W.N., Kane, F.D., et al. An investigation of the relation between life experience, personality characteristics, and general susceptibility to illness. *Psychosomatic Medicine.* 1958; 20(4): 278–295.

23. Hinkle, L.E., Wolff, H.G. Ecological investigations of the relationship between illness, life experience and the social environment. *Annals of Internal Medicine.* 1958; 29: 1373–1388.

24. Hinkle, L.E. Studies of human ecology in relation to health and behavior. *BioScience.* August 1965; 517–520.

25. Justice, B., op. cit., 67.

26. These studies are reviewed in Dreher, H. *Mind-Body Unity: A New Vision for Mind-Body Science and Medicine* (Baltimore: The Johns Hopkins University Press, 2003), 59–60.

27. Seligman, M.E.P., op. cit., 172–174.

28. Seligman, M.E.P., op. cit., 174.

29. Ornish, D. *Love and Survival: The Scientific Basis for the Healing Power of Intimacy* (New York: HarperPerennial), 1999.

30. Randomized trial of knee arthroscopy (study finds common knee surgery no better than placebo). Baylor College of Medicine, Office of Public Affairs. www.bcm.edu/pa/kneeqa.htm (accessed January 20, 2005).

31. Finch, E.E., Tanzi, R.E. Genetics of aging. *Science.* 1997; 278(5337): 407–411.

32. Disabilities decline among elderly. *Amarillo Business Journal.* http://businessjournal.net/stories/042897/health.html (accessed January 20, 2005).

33. Hurdle, J. Lose weight, stay active, prevent Alzheimer's—Studies. Reuters Online. http://www.reuters.com. July 19, 2004 (accessed July 20, 2004).

34. McCullough, M.E., Hoyt, W.T., Larson, D.B., Koenig, H., Thoresen, C. Religious involvement and mortality: A meta-analytic review. *Health Psychology.* 2000; 19(3): 211–222.

35. Idler, E., Kasl, S. Health perceptions and survival: do global evaluations of health really predict mortality? *Journal of Gerontology.* 1991; 46(2): S55–65.

36. Justice, B., op. cit., 139.

37. Finch, E.E., Tanzi, R.E., op. cit., 407.

38. Schleifer, S.J., Keller, S.E., Camerino, J.C., et al. Suppression of lymphocyte stimulation following bereavement. *Journal of the American Medical Association.* 1983; 250:3: 374–377.

39. Kamen-Siegel, L., Rodin, J., Seligman, M.E.P., Dwyer, J. Explanatory style and cell-mediated immunity in elderly men and women. *Health Psychology.* 1991; 10(4): 229–235.

40. Buchanan, G.M., Seligman, M.E.P., eds. *Explanatory Style* (Hillsdale: Lawrence Erlbaum Associates, Inc, 1995).

41. Baumeister R.F. *Evil: Inside Human Violence and Cruelty* (San Francisco: W.H. Freeman; 1999), 135–148.

42. Baumeister, R.F., Smart, L., Boden, J.M. Relationship of threatened egotism to violence and aggression: the dark side of high self-esteem. *Psychological Review.* 1996; 103: 5–33.

43. Baumeister, R.F., *Evil*, 25.

44. Baumeister, R.F., ibid., 384.

45. Begley, S. You're OK, I'm terrific: unjustified feelings of self-worth cause aggression. *Wall Street Journal.* July 13, 1998. www.wsj.com (accessed July 28, 1998).

46. Seligman, M.E.P., op. cit., 205–234.

47. Ibid., 182–184.

48. Ibid., ix.

49. Dreher, H. *Mind-Body Unity: A New Vision for Mind-Body Science and Medicine* (Baltimore: The Johns Hopkins University Press, 2003), 60.

50. Dreher, H., ibid., 60.

51. Ibid., 41–42.

52. Ibid., 61.

53. Justice, B., op. cit., 293–294.

54. Williams, S.V., Williams, R. *Lifeskills* (New York: Random House, 1997), 268–70.

55. Justice, B., op. cit., 148.

56. *Webster's New Explorer Dictionary of Quotations*, s.v. "Feiffer, Jules."

57. Gardner, J.W. *Excellence* (New York: W.W. Norton, 1995).

58. Lowell, R. "If we see light at the end of the tunnel, /It's the light of the oncoming train." From the poem: "Since 1939." In *Day by Day* (New York: Farrar, Straus, Giroux, 1978).

59. *Webster's New Explorer Dictionary of Quotations*, s.v. "Stevenson, Adlai."

60. www.heartsandminds.org/poverty/hungerfacts.htm (accessed January 19, 2004).

61. *New York Times.* "America's promises." Editorial. January 28, 2005, A20.

2. Forgetting

1. Azar, B. Why men lose keys—and women find them. *American Psychological Association Monitor.* August 1996: 32.

2. Ibid.

3. Ibid.

4. "Brain activity study concludes men are better at navigating." May 29, 2001. www.ananova.com (accessed May 30, 2001).

5. "Don't make rude gestures at traffic cameras!" October 13, 2000. http://dailynews.yahoo.com (accessed October 14, 2000).

6. Melechi, A. Senses and sensibility. Sidebar: The memory man (or the man who couldn't forget). *Fortean Times.* August 1998; 113: 28–31.

7. Luria, A.L. *The Mind of a Mnemonist.* L. Solotaroff, trans. (New York: Basic Books, 1968).

8. Arkes, H.R., Wortmann, R.L., Saville, P.D., Harkness, A.R. Hindsight bias among physicians weighting the likelihood of diagnoses. *Journal of Applied Psychology.* 1981; 66: 252–54.

9. Hawkins, S.A., Hastie, R. Hindsight: Biased judgments of past events after the outcomes are known. *Psychological Bulletin.* 1990; 107: 311–27.

10. Hastie, R., Schkade, D.A., Payne, J.W. Juror judgments in civil cases: Hindsight effects on judgments of liability for punitive damages. *Law and Human Behavior.* 1999; 23: 597–614.

11. Reuters. "Octopus opens jam jar in one minute." June 1, 2000. http://dailynews.yahoo.com (accessed June 2, 2000).

12. Netting, J. Memory may draw addicts back to cocaine. *Science News.* May 12, 2001; 159 (19): 292.

13. Vorel, S.R., Gardner, E.L., et al. Relapse to cocaine-seeking after hippocampal theta burst stimulation. *Science.* 2001; 292: 1175.

14. Pettingale, K.W. The biological correlates of psychological responses to cancer. *Journal of Psychosomatic Research.* 1981; 25: 453–458.

15. Taylor, S. *Positive Illusions: Creative Self-deception and the Healthy Mind* (New York: Basic Books, 1989), 131.

16. Ibid., 227–228.

17. Ibid., 229.

18. Feedback. *New Scientist.* December 5, 1998.

19. Schacter, D.L. *The Seven Sins of Memory* (New York: Houghton Mifflin, 2001), 161–162, 167–168.

20. D'Amato, G. Van de Velde still smiling after British fiasco. *Milwaukee Journal Sentinel.* August 12, 1999: 1.

21. Mineka, S., Nugent, K. Mood-congruent memory biases in anxiety and depression. In D.L. Schacter, ed. *Memory Distortion: How Minds, Brains, and Societies Reconstruct the Past* (Cambridge, Mass.: Harvard University Press, 1995), 173–96.

22. Shay, J. *Achilles in Vietnam: Combat Trauma and the Undoing of Character* (New York: Atheneum, 1994), 50.

23. *The Viking Book of Aphorisms.* Auden, W.H. and Kronenberger, L., eds. (New York: Barnes & Noble, 1993), 361.

24. Carroll, L. *Curiosa Mathematica* (New York: Classic Books, 2000.)

25. Freyd, J.J. *Betrayal Trauma: The Logic of Forgetting Childhood Abuse* (Cambridge, Mass.: Harvard University Press, 1996), 60–78.

26. Bower, B. Repression tries for experimental comeback. *Science News.* March 17, 2001; 159: 184.

27. Wenzlaff, R.M., Wegner, D.M. Thought suppression. *Annual Review of Psychology.* 2000; 51: 59–91.

28. Mitka, M. Aging patients are advised "stay active to stay alert." *Journal of the American Medical Association.* 2001; 285(19): 2437–2438.

29. Fillit, H.M., Butler, R.N., O'Connell, A.W., Albert, M.S., et al. Achieving and maintaining cognitive vitality with aging. *Mayo Clinic Proceedings,* 2002; 77(7): 681–96. Available at: http://nootropics.com/aging/ (accessed April 20, 2005).

30. Tang, Y.P., et al. Genetic enhancement of learning and memory in mice. *Nature.* 1999; 401: 63–69.

31. Tully, T. Quoted in Weiner, J. *Time, Love, Memory: A Great Biologist and His Quest for the Origins of Behavior* (New York: Alfred A. Knopf, 1999), 29.

32. Levin, J. *God, Faith, and Health* (New York: John Wiley, 2001), 23–27.

33. Koenig, H.G., McCullough, M.E., Larson, D.B. *Handbook of Religion and Health* (New York: Oxford University Press, 2001), 271.

34. Levinson, A. Two-time memory champion still lives by Post-Its. *San Antonio Express-News.* February 22, 1999: 5A.

35. Schacter, D.L., op. cit., 34–36. Schacter describes mnemonic devices that rely on visual imagery, as well as various commercial programs and products designed to enhance memory and retention—which ones work and which ones don't.

36. Keegan, J. *The Mask of Command* (New York: Viking, 1987), 136.

37. *The Viking Book of Aphorisms,* 360.

3. Novelty

1. Baars, B.J. I.P. Pavlov and the freedom reflex. *Journal of Consciousness Studies.* 2003; 10(11): 19–40.

2. Laming, D. *The Measurement of Sensation* (New York: Oxford University Press, 1997).

3. Baars, B.J., op. cit., 23.

4. Blazer, A.N. *Santana: War Chief of the Mescalero Apache.* Pruitt, A.R., ed. (Taos, NM: Dog Soldier Press, 1999), 190–191, 282.

5. Kasamatsu, A., Hirai, T. An EEG study of Zen meditation. *Folia Psychiatrica et Neurologia Japonica.* 1966; 20: 315–336. Reprinted in Tart, Charles T., ed. *Altered States of Consciousness.* 3rd ed. (New York: HarperCollins, 501–14).

6. Kesten, D. *Feeding the Body, Nourishing the Soul* (Berkeley, Calif.: Conari Press, 1997).

7. Kesten, D. *The Healing Secrets of Food* (Novato, Calif.: New World Library, 2001).

8. Honoré, C. *In Praise of Slowness* (San Francisco: HarperSanFrancisco, 2004).

9. Fear of new things shortens life. www.NewScientist.com (accessed December 8, 2003).

10. Dossey, L. The case for nonlocality. *Reinventing Medicine* (San Francisco: HarperSanFrancisco, 1999).

11. Jonas, W.B., Crawford, C.C. *Healing, Intention and Energy Medicine: Scientific Research Methods and Clinical Applications* (New York: Churchill Livingstone, 2003), xv–xix.

12. Crawford, C.C., Sparber, A.G., Jonas, W.B. A systematic review of the quality of research on hands-on healing: clinical and laboratory studies. *Alternative Therapies in Health and Medicine.* 2003: 9(3): A96–A104.

13. Foucault, Jean-Bernard-Léon. *Encyclopædia Britannica.* www.britannica.com/eb/article?tocId=9035012 (accessed April 20, 2005).

14. Von Helmholtz, H. Quoted in Murphy, M. *The Future of the Body* (Los Angeles: Jeremy P. Tarcher, 1992), 345.

15. Targ, R., Puthoff, H. *Mind-Reach. Scientists Look at Psychic Ability* (New York: Delta, 1977), 169. Also: Scanning the issue [editorial]. *Proceedings of the IEEE,* March 1976); LXIV(3): 291.

16. Radin, D. *The Conscious Universe* (San Francisco: HarperSanFrancisco, 1997), 1.

17. *The Viking Book of Aphorisms,* Auden, W.H. and Kronenberger, L., eds. (New York: Barnes & Noble, 1993), 104.

18. Hurdle, J. Lose weight, stay active, prevent Alzheimer's—studies. www.reutershealth.com/en/index.html. July 10, 2004 (accessed October 21, 2004).

19. Bierce, A. *The Devil's Dictionary* (New York: Oxford University Press, 1999).

4. Tears

1. Furlow, B. The uses of crying and begging animal behavior. *Natural History.* October 2000. www.findarticles.com/p/articles/mi_m1134/is_8_109/ai_65913174 (accessed July 19, 2004).

2. Ibid.

3. Solter, A. Crying for comfort: distressed babies need to be held. *Mothering.* January-February 2004. www.mothering.com/9-0-0/html/9-1-0/crying-for-comfort.shtml (accessed July 19, 2004).

4. Watson, J.B. Quoted in Balbus, I. D., *Emotional Rescue: The Theory and Practice of a Feminist Father* (New York: Routledge, 1998), 83.

5. Holt, L.E. Quoted in Balbus, I. D., op. cit., 83.

6. Spock, B. *Dr. Spock's Baby and Child Care.* 8th ed. (New York: Pocket, 2004).

7. McCardell, E. Review of *Adult Crying: A Biopsychosocial Approach.* Edited by Vingerhoets, A., and Cornelius, R.R. *Human Nature Review.* 2002; 3: 219–221. human-nature.com/nibbs/03/crying.html (accessed July 19, 2004).

8. Downey, C. Toxic tears: how crying keeps you healthy. community.healthgate. com/GetContent.asp?siteid=ucsd&docid=/healthy/mind/2000/crying/index (accessed July 21, 2004).

9. Ibid.

10. Foreman, J. Sob story: why we cry, and how. *Boston Globe.* October 21, 1996: CI. www.boston.com/globe/search/stories/health/health_sense/102196.htm.

11. www.lachrymatory.com, www.tearcatcher.com, and www.morrae.com/tears/ (accessed July 19, 2004).

12. LePage, K.E., Schafer, D.W., Miller, A. Alternating unilateral lachrymation. *American Journal of Clinical Hypnosis.* 1992; 34(4): 255–260.

13. LePage, K.E., Schafer, D.W. Alternating unilateral lachrymations as therapeutic cleansing and healing in a case of child sexual abuse. *Hypnos.* 2000; XXVII: 171–179.

14. Foreman, J., op. cit.

15. Frey, W.H. *Crying: The Mystery of Tears* (New York: HarperCollins, 1985).

16. Frey II, W. Quoted in Downey, C. Toxic tears: how crying keeps you healthy. http://community.healthgate.com/GetContent.asp?siteid=ucsd&docid=/ healthy/mind/2000/crying/index (accessed July 21, 2004).

17. Bernfeld, B.M. Quoted in Downey, C. Toxic tears: how crying keeps you healthy. community.healthgate.com/GetContent.asp?siteid=ucsd&docid=/healthy/ mind/2000/crying/index (accessed July 21, 2004).

18. Gross, J. Quoted in Holladay, A. People may weep for help. November 28, 2001. www.usatoday.com/news/science/wonderquest/2001-11-28-weep.htm (accessed July 21, 2004).

19. Holladay, A. People may weep for help. November 28, 2001. www. usatoday.com/news/science/wonderquest/2001-11-28-weep.htm (accessed July 21, 2004).

20. Murube, J., Murube, L., Murube, A. Origin and types of emotional tearing. *European Journal of Ophthalmology.* 1999; 9(2): 77–84.

21. Ishii, H., Nagashima, M., Tanno, M., Nakajima, A., Yoshino, S. Does being easily moved to tears as a response to psychological stress reflect response to treatment and the general prognosis in patients with rheumatoid arthritis? *Clinical and Experimental Rheumatology.* 2003; 21(5): 611–616.

22. Cousins, N. *Anatomy of an Illness* (New York: W.W. Norton, 1979).

23. Cousins, N. Anatomy of an illness (as perceived by the patient). *New England Journal of Medicine.* 1976; 295(26): 1458–1463.

24. Wagner, R.E., Hexel, M., Bauer, W.W., Kropiunigg, U. Crying in hospitals: a survey of doctors', nurses', and medical students' experience and attitudes. *Medical Journal of Australia.* 1997; 166(1): 13–16. www.ncbi.nlm.nih.gov/entrez/query. fcgi?cmd=Retrieve&db=pubmed&dopt=Abstract&list_uids=9006606 (accessed July 21, 2004).

25. Riemann, R., Pfennigsdorf, S., Riemann, E., Naumann, M. Successful treatment of crocodile tears by injection of botulinum toxin into the lacrimal gland: a case report. *Ophthalmology.* 1999; 106(12): 2322–2324.

26. Hofmann, R.J. Treatment of Frey's syndrome (gustatory sweating) and "crocodile tears" (gustatory epiphora) with purified botulinum toxin. *Opthalmologic, Plastic, and Reconstructive Surgery.* 2000; 16(4): 289–291.

27. Gutman, C. Botulinum toxin injection controls crocodile tears. June 1, 2002. www.escrs.org/eurotimes/June%202002/botulinum.asp (accessed July 21, 2004).

28. Botox to curb sweating. July 21, 2004. www.news24.com/News24/Technology/News/0,,2-13-1443_1560572,00.html (accessed July 21, 2004).

29. FDA okays Botox for sweating. July 20, 2004. money.cnn.com/2004/07/20/news/midcaps/botox_sweat.reut/ (accessed July 21, 2004).

30. Virani, M.J., Jain, S. Trigeminal schwannoma associated with pathological laughter and crying. *Neurology India.* 2001; 49: 162–5. www.neurologyindia.com/article.asp?issn=0028-3886;year=2001;volume=49;issue=2;spage=162;epage=5;aulast=Virani (accessed July 22, 2004).

31. Anderson, G., Vesterguard, K., Rils, J.O. Post-stroke pathological crying treated with the selective serotonin reuptake inhibitor, citalopram. *Lancet.* 1993; 342: 837–839.

32. Franklin, B. Quoted in About onions: quotes. Website of the National Onion Association. www.onions-usa.org/about/quotes.asp (accessed July 22, 2004).

33. Imai, S. An onion enzyme that makes the eyes water. *Nature.* 2002; 419685. dx.doi.org/10.1038/419685a.

34. Block, E. Quoted in Pickrell, J. Less crying in the kitchen: tasty, tearfree onions on the horizon. *Science News.* 2002; 162(16). www.sciencenews.org/articles/20021019/fob3.asp (accessed July 22, 2004).

35. Web site of the National Onion Association. www.onions-usa.org/about/history.asp (accessed July 22, 2004).

36. *Webster's New World Dictionary.* 2nd College ed.

37. Web site of the National Onion Association. www.onions-usa.org/about/quotes.asp (accessed July 22, 2004).

38. Ibid.

5. Dirt

1. Hamilton, G. Let them eat dirt. *New Scientist.* July 18, 1998;159 (2143): 26–31.

2. Pickover, C.A. *Strange Brains and Genius* (New York: HarperCollins, 1998), 292–293.

3. Ibid.

4. Hamilton, G., op. cit., 26.

5. Dossey, L. *Healing Words: The Power of Prayer and the Practice of Medicine* (San Francisco: HarperSanFrancisco, 1993).

6. Tomes, N. *The Gospel of Germs: Men, Women, and the Microbe in American Life* (Cambridge, Mass.: Harvard University Press, 1998), 33.

7. Bynum, W.F. Darwin and the doctors: Evolution, diathesis, and germs in nineteenth-century Britain. *Gesnerus*; 1983; 40: 43–53.

8. Theodore Roosevelt Collection, Houghton Library, Harvard University, Cambridge, Mass.

9. Tomes, N., op. cit., 25.

10. Condran, G. Changing patterns of epidemic disease in New York City. *Hives of Sickness: Public Health and Epidemics in New York City.* David Rosner, ed. (New Brunswick, N.J.: Rutgers University Press, 1995), 27–41.

11. Interview 1-4-A. Oral Histories, Corinne Krause Collection, Library and Archives, Historical Society of Western Pennsylvania, Pittsburgh, Penn.

12. Making Cellophane Conscious. Scrapbook, 1932–1933, Records of the Du Pont Cellophane Company, Series 2, Part 2, Archives of the E.I. Du Pont de Nemours and Company, Hagley Museum and Library, Wilmington, Del.

13. Marchand, R. *Advertising the American Dream. Making Way for Modernity, 1920–1940* (Berkeley, Calif.: University of California Press, 1985), 18–21.

14. Calver, H.N. Foreword. *Regulatory Measures Concerning the Prohibition of the Common Drinking Cup and the Sterilization of Eating and Drinking Utensils in Public Places* (New York: Public Health Committee, Cup and Container Institute, 1936), 3.

15. Parker, W.M. The hygiene of the holy communion. *Medical Record.* 41; 1892: 264–265. Minutes of the General Assembly of the Presbyterian Church in the United States of America. 1895; 18:75. Department of History, Presbyterian Church (U.S.A.), Philadelphia.

16. Anders, H.S. The progress of the individual cup movement, especially among churches. *Journal of the American Medical Association.* 1897; 29: 789–794.

17. Hamilton, G., op. cit., 27.

18. Hamilton, G., op. cit., 28.

19. Strachan, D.P. Hay fever, hygiene and household size. *British Medical Journal.* 1989; 299: 1259–1260.

20. Ibid.

21. Shahben, S.O., Aaby, P., Hall, A.J., et al. Measles and atopy in Guinea-Bissau. *Lancet.* 1996; 347: 1792.

22. Aaby, P., Samb, B., Simondon, F., Seck, A.M., Knudsen, K., Whittle, H. Non-specific beneficial effect of measles immunisation: analysis of mortality studies from developing countries. *British Medical Journal.* 1995; 311: 481

23. Hamilton, G., op. cit., 28.

24. Hamilton, G., op. cit., 29.

25. Ponsonby, A., van der Mei, I., Dwyer, T., et al. Exposure to infant siblings during early life and risk of multiple sclerosis. *Journal of the American Medical Association.* 2005; 293(4): 463–469.

26. Leibowitz, U., Antonovsky, A., Medalie, J., Smith, H.A., Halpern, L., Alter, M. Epidemiological study of multiple sclerosis in Israel, II: multiple sclerosis and level of sanitation. *Journal of Neurological and Neurosurgical Psychiatry.* 1966; 29: 60–68.

27. Hamilton, G., op. cit., 30.

28. Wang, C.-C., Rook, G.A.W. Inhibition of an established allergic response to ovalbumin in BALB/c mice by killed *Mycobacterium vaccae. Immunology.* 1998; 93: 307–313.

29. Hamilton, G., op. cit., 30.

30. Ibid.

31. Hamilton, G., op. cit., 31.

32. Ibid.

33. *Webster's New World Dictionary.* 2nd College ed.

34. Horgan, P. *Great River: The Rio Grande in North American History* (Hanover, N.H.: University Press of New England/Wesleyan University Press, 1984), 48, 222, 224.

35. Sardello, R. *Facing the Soul with Soul* (Hudson, N.Y.: Lindisfarne Press, 1992), 163.

36. Estés, C.P. *Women Who Run with the Wolves* (New York: Ballantine, 1992), 335.

37. Ibid.

38. Ibid.

39. Jung, C.G. On the psychology of the trickster figure. In Radin, *The Trickster: A Study in American Indian Mythology* (New York: Schocken, 1972), 197.

40. Dossey, L. The trickster: medicine's forgotten character. *Alternative Therapies in Health and Medicine.* 1996; 2 (2): 6–14.

41. Taylor, E. Interview by Bonnie Horrigan. *Alternative Therapies in Health and Medicine.* 1998: 4 (6): 79–87.

42. Duff, K. *The Alchemy of Illness* (New York: Pantheon, 1993), 88–89.

43. Ibid., 61.

44. Jung, C.G. *Vision Seminars: From the Complete Notes of Mary Foote* (Zurich, Switzerland: Spring Publications, 1976), 136.

45. Bayles, M. Attributed.

46. *Bartlett's Familiar Quotations*, 16th ed., s.v. "Diogenes."

6. Music

1. "In our Western music we still know the modes 'major' and 'minor.' The Greeks had five modes, known to us by their names—Ionian, Aeolian, Lydian, Dorian, and Phrygian—which referred also to ethnic groupings within Greece. Each of these modes, each of which had submodes, was easily recognized by listeners, and each created a characteristic mood, just as we might say, 'That sounded like a Scottish ballad. This sounds like a Spanish dance.' Each Greek mode was constructed from an invariable sequence of relationships between the notes that no other mode possessed. . . . The Dorian was martial, the Phrygian engendered contentment, . . . the Ionian softly alluring, apparently making seduction easier." Thomas Cahill, *Sailing the Wine-Dark Sea: Why the Greeks Matter* (New York: Nan A. Talese/Doubleday, 2003), 87.

2. Linton, M. The Mozart effect. *First Things*. March 1999: 10–13.

3. *The Viking Book of Aphorisms*. Auden, W.H., and Kronenberger, L., eds. (New York: Barnes & Noble; 1993), 289.

4. Taruskin, R. Music's dangers and the case for control. *The New York Times*. December 9, 2001; Section 2, p. 1, 36.

5. Labi, N. Rhythmless nation. *Time*. Fall 2001 special issue: 44.

6. Korpe, M. Quoted in Labi, N. Rhythmless nation. *Time*. Fall 2001 special issue: 44.

7. Taruskin, R., op. cit., 1.

8. *Bartlett's Familiar Quotations*, 16th ed., s.v. "Pope, Alexander."

9. Taruskin, R., op. cit., 1, 36.

10. Cohen, A. All you need is hate. *Time*. Fall 2001 special issue: 46.

11. Cured by carols. *Fortean Times*. June 2000; 136: 22.

12. Ibid.

13. Aldridge, D. Philosophical speculations on two therapeutic applications of breath. *Subtle Energies & Energy Medicine*. 2002; 12(12): 107–124.

14. Marwick, C. Music hath charms for care of preemies. *Journal of the American Medical Association*. 2000; 283(4): 468–469.

15. Hirschfield, R. The lullaby cure. *Discover*. June 2000: 26.

16. Standley, J.M. A meta-analysis of the efficacy of music therapy for premature infants. *Journal of Pediatric Nursing*. 2002; 12: 107–113.

17. Standley, J.M. The effect of contingent music to increase non-nutritive sucking of premature infants. *Journal of Pediatric Nursing.* 2000; 5: 493–495, 498–499.

18. Standley J.M. The effect of music and multimodal stimulation on responses of premature infants in neonatal intensive care. *Journal of Pediatric Nursing.* 1998; 6: 532–538.

19. Standley, J.M. Therapeutic effects of music and mother's voice on premature infants. *Journal of Pediatric Nursing.* 1995; 6: 509–512, 574.

20. Musical pacifiers. Research in Review. Florida State University; Fall and Winter, 1999. researchback.magnet.fsu.edu/researchr/fallwinter99/departments/abstracts/ab_musical.html (accessed December 27, 2002).

21. Maniscalco, M., et al., Nasal nitric oxide measurements before and after repeated humming maneuvers. *European Journal of Clinical Investigation.* 2003; 33(12): 1090–1094.

22. What is nitric oxide? ase.tufts.edu/biology/Firefly/#Nitric (accessed January 3, 2004).

23. Weitzberg, E., Lundberg, J.O. Humming greatly increases nasal nitric oxide. *American Journal of Respiratory and Critical Care Medicine.* 2002; 166(2): 131–132.

24. Purce, J. *The Mystic Spiral* (London: Thames and Hudson, 1974). www.jillpurce.com/about_main.htm.

25. Green, M.F., Kinsbourne, M. Subvocal activity and auditory hallucinations: clues for behavioral treatments? *Schizophrenia Bulletin.* 1990; 16(4): 617–625.

26. Green, M.F., Kinsbourne, M. Auditory hallucinations in schizophrenia: does humming help? *Biological Psychiatry.* 1990; 27(8): 934–935.

27. Campbell, D. *The Mozart Effect* (New York: Avon, 1997).

28. Ibid., 256.

29. Keyes, L.E. *Toning: The Creative Power of the Voice* (Marina del Rey, Calif.: DeVorss & Co., 1973).

30. Harrison, D. Revealed: how purrs are secret to cats' nine lives. www.telegraph.co.uk. Issue 2123, Sunday March 18, 2001 (accessed March 18, 2001).

31. Gordon, L.E., Thacher, C., Kapatkin, A. High-rise syndrome in dogs: 81 cases (1985–1991). *Journal of the American Veterinary Medical Association.* 1993; 202(1): 118–22.

32. Harrison, D., op. cit.

33. Gregorios, P. M. *Cosmic Man: The Divine Presence. The Theology of Gregory of Nyssa* (New York: Paragon, 1988), 13.

34. Thomas, L. *The Medusa and the Snail* (New York: Penguin, 1995), 16–17.

35. Scientist tunes in to gene compositions. San Jose *Mercury News.* May 13, 1986: E1.

36. Whitehouse, D. Listen to your DNA. BBC News Online. November 26, 1998. news.bbc.co.uk/hi/english/sci/tech/newsid_222000/222591.stm (accessed July 7, 2002).

37. Ibid.

38. Greenman, C. Now, follow the bouncing nucleotide. *The New York Times* Web site. September 13, 2001. www.nytimes.com (accessed January 2, 2003).

39. Dunn, J., Clark, M.A. Life music: the sonification of proteins. December 15, 1997. Web site: Leonardo On-Line. mitpress2.mit.edu/e-journals/Leonardo/isast/articles/lifemusic.html (accessed January 2, 2003).

40. Whitehouse, D. Listening to geometry. BBC News Online. December 14, 1998. news.bbc.co.uk/hi/english/sci/tech/newsid_128000/128906.stm (accessed January 2, 2003).

41. Ibid.

42. Stewart I. *The Collapse of Chaos: Discovering Simplicity in a Complex World* (New York: Penguin, 1994).

43. Ibid.

44. Whitehead, D., op. cit.

45. Nollman, J. Water song. *Resurgence.* July–August 2001; 207: 21.

46. Ibid.

47. Hogan, J. Dunes alive with the sand of music. *New Scientist.* December 18, 2004; 184 (2478): 8.

48. Andreotti, B., loc. cit., 8.

49. Allen, K., Blascovich, J. Effects of music on cardiovascular reactivity among surgeons. *Journal of the American Medical Association.* 1994; 272(11): 882–884.

50. Nietzsche, F. Quoted in Levy, O. (ed.) *The Twilight of the Idols* (New York: Russell and Russell, 1964), 16:6.

51. Kumar, A.M., et al. Music therapy increases serum melatonin levels in patients with Alzheimer's disease. *Alternative Therapies in Health and Medicine.* 1999; 5(6): 49–57.

52. Kumar, A. Quoted in Vail, J. Music therapy helps Alzheimer's patients. January 28, 2000. http://dailynews.yahoo.com (accessed January 29, 2000).

53. Kumar, A.M., loc. cit., 56.

54. Milius, S. Cardinal girls learn faster than boys. *Science News.* June 9, 2001; 159: 365.

55. Jacobs, G.D. *The Ancestral Mind* (New York: Penguin, 2003), 150.

56. Gray, P. The music of nature and the nature of music. *Science.* 2001; 291: 52–56.

57. Chandler, D. Ancient note: music as a bridge between the species. *The Boston Globe.* January 5, 2001.

58. Cook, G. Wired for sound. *The Boston Globe.* April 15, 2001, 6–7.

59. Jacobs, G.D., loc. cit.

60. Shaw, G., Rauscher, F. Listening to Mozart enhances spatial-temporal reasoning. *Nature.* 1993; 365: 611.

61. Rauscher, F.H., Shaw, G.L., Ky, K.N. Listening to Mozart enhances spatial-temporal reasoning: towards a neurophysiological basis. *Neuroscience Letters.* 1995; 185: 44–47.

62. Steele, K.M., Brown, J.D., Stoecker, J.A. Failure to confirm the Rauscher and Shaw description of recovery of the Mozart effect. *Perceptual and Motor Skills.* 1999; 88(3 Pt. 1): 843–848.

63. McCutcheon, L.E. Another failure to generalize the Mozart effect. *Psychological Reports.* 2000; 87(1): 325–330.

64. Campbell, D. *The Mozart Effect* (New York: Avon, 1997). www.mozarteffect. com.

65. Thompson, B.M., Andrews, S.R. An historical commentary on the physiological effects of music: Tomatis, Mozart and neurophysiology. *Integrative Physiology and Behavioral Science.* 2000; 35(3): 174–188.

66. *Bartlett's Familiar Quotations,* 16th ed, s.v. "Flaubert."

67. Riemer, J. Heavenly music on earth. www.ug.bcc.bilkent.edu.tr/~mcaliska/ perlman.html. Also available at: SchwartzReport. April 15, 2001. www. stephanschwartz.com (acccessed December 28, 2002).

68. Ibid.

69. Michael Toms, ed. *Wise Words* (Carlsbad, Calif.: Hay House, 1998). Quote for November 22, 1998.

70. *The Santa Fe Opera 2002 Festival Season* (Santa Fe, N.M.: Santa Fe Opera, 2002), 1.

71. Mingus, C., attributed.

72. Travis, J. Crystal listens for telltale sound of virus. *Science News.* 2001; 160: 134.

73. Behar, M. Hears to your health. *Scientific American.* 2002; 286 (3): 20–21.

74. Corliss, W.R. The music of the genes. Science Frontiers Online. December, 28, 2002. www.science-frontiers.com/sf046/sf046p08.htm (accessed December, 28, 2002).

75. Whitehouse, D. Listen to your DNA. BBC News Online. November 26, 1998. news.bbc.co.uk/hi/english/sci/tech/newsid_222000/222591.stm (accessed July 7, 2002).

76. Klinkenborg, V. Hearing the echo of earthly music. www.nytimes. com/2001/01/17/opinion/17WED3.html (accessed January 17, 2001).

77. Fabian, A.C., Sanders, J.S., Allen, S.W., Crawford, C.S., Iwasawa, K., Johnstone, R.M., Schmidt, R.W., Taylor, G.B. A deep *Chandra* observation of the

Perseus cluster: shocks and ripples. *Monthly Notices of the Royal Astronomical Society.* September 2003: L43–L47. www-xray.ast.cam.ac.uk/papers/per_200ks.pdf.

78. Cowen, R. A low note in the cosmos. *Science News.* September 13, 2003; 164(11): 163. www.sciencenews.org/20030405/fob7.asp.

79. Music of the spheres in B-flat. *USA Today.* September 10, 2003: 1.

7. Risk

1. Keyes, R. *Chancing It: Why We Take Risks* (Boston, Mass.: Little, Brown, 1985), 273.

2. Rachman, S.J. *Fear and Courage* (San Francisco: W.H. Freeman, 1978), 27–42.

3. Watson, P. *War on the Mind: The Military Uses and Abuses of Psychology* (New York: Basic Books, 1978), 218–220.

4. SchwartzReport. Stephan A. Schwartz, editor. www.schwartzreport.net. August 29, 2000.

5. Koestler, A. *Janus: A Summing Up* (New York: Random House, 1978), 266.

6. Bower, B. 9/11's fatal road toll. *Science News.* January 17, 2004; 165: 37–38.

7. Spencer, J., Crossen, C. Why do Americans believe danger lurks everywhere? How a fixation on risk, fed by labs, law and media, haunts world's safest nation. *Wall Street Journal.* April 24, 2003. (accessed July 20, 2003): www.jefferyscottmitchell.com/Images/raw/why_are_americans_so_scared.htm.

8. Granger, D.A., Booth, A., Johnson, D.R. Human aggression and enumerative measures of immunity. *Psychosomatic Medicine.* 2000; 62(4): 583–590.

9. Justice, B. *Who Gets Sick: How Beliefs, Moods, and Thoughts Affect Your Health* (Houston: Peak Press, 2000), 206–7.

10. Hazuda, H. Women's employment status and their risks for chronic disease. Colloquium presentation, University of Texas School of Public Health, Houston, Texas. March 1984.

11. Waldron, I., Herold, J. Employment, attitudes toward employment, and women's health. Presentation at the annual meeting of the Society of Behavioral Medicine, Philadelphia, PA, May 1984.

12. Pietromonaco, P.R., Manis, J., Frohart-Lane, K. Psychological consequences of multiple social roles. Paper presented at the annual meeting of the American Psychological Association, Toronto, August 1984.

13. Unruh, Jr., J.D. *The Plains Across* (Urbana: University of Illinois Press, 1979), 408–413.

14. Billington, R.A. *America's Frontier Heritage* (New York: Holt, Rinehart and Winston, 1966), 32.

15. Hollon, W.E. *Frontier Violence: Another Look* (New York: Oxford University Press, 1974), 196, 211.

16. Keyes, R., op. cit., 267.

17. Keyes, R., loc. cit., 270.

18. Keyes, R., loc. cit., 271.

19. www.outwardbound.com (accessed July 20, 2003).

20. Keyes, R., loc. cit., 41–51.

21. Keyes, R., loc. cit., 274.

22. Keyes, R., loc. cit., 280.

23. Piliavin, J.A., et al. *Journal of Personality and Social Psychology.* 1982; 43: 1200–1213.

24. Blachly, P.H. Commentary. *Life-Threatening Behavior.* 1971; 1: 5–9.

25. Phillips, H. Teens may go where adults fear to tread. *New Scientist.* 4 December, 2004; 184(2476): 8.

26. Clare, A. It isn't the hormones. SchwartzReport. July 31, 2000. www.schwartzreport.net. See also Anthony Clare, *On Men: Masculinity in Crisis* (London: Chatto & Windus, 2000).

27. Zuckerman, M. Are you a risk taker? *Psychology Today.* November 2000. www.findarticles.com (accessed July 27, 2003).

28. Coniff, R. Why we take risks. *Discover.* December 2001; 62–67.

29. Explorer heroes. myhero.com/hero.asp?hero=stevefossett (accessed July 27, 2003).

30. The *Challenger* disaster 10 years later. *Life.* January 26, 1996. www.life.com/Life/space/challenger/challenger06.html (accessed July 27, 2003).

31. Koenig, H.G., Idler, E., Kasl, S., Hays, J.C., George, L.K., Musick, M., Larson, D.B., Collins, T.R., Benson, H. Religion, spirituality, and medicine: A rebuttal to skeptics. *International Journal of Psychiatry and Medicine.* 1999; 29(2): 123–131.

32. Levin, J. *God, Faith, and Health* (New York: John Wiley & Sons, 2001).

33. Levin, J.S. Religion and health: Is there an association, is it valid, and is it causal? *Social Science and Medicine.* 1994; 38: 1475–1482.

34. Dossey, L. The case for nonlocality. *Reinventing Medicine* (San Francisco: HarperSanFrancisco, 1999), 37–84.

35. Benor, D.J. *Spiritual Healing* (Southfield, Mich.: Vision, 2002).

36. Kennedy, J.E., Abbott, R.A., Rosenberg, B.S. Changes in spirituality and well-being in a retreat program for cardiac patients. *Alternative Therapies in Health and Medicine.* 2002; 8(4): 64–73.

37. Koenig, H.G. Impact of belief on immune function. *Modern Aspects of Immunology.* 2001; 1(5): 187–190.

38. Stein, J. Just say om. *Time.* July 27, 2003. Source: www.time.com/time/magazine/printout/0,8816,471136,00.html (accessed July 29, 2003.

39. Bray, R.S. *Armies of Pestilence* (New York: Barnes & Noble, 1998), 131.

40. Hope-Ross, M., Travers, S., Mooney, D. Solar retinopathy following religious rituals. *Br J Ophthalmol.* 1998; 72(12): 931–934.

41. Khogali, M. Epidemiology of heat illness during the Makkah pilgrimages in Saudi Arabia. *Int J Epidemiol.* 1983; 12(3): 267–273.

42. Zenkert-Andersson, K., Hedeland, H., Manhem, P. Too little exposure to sun may cause vitamin D deficiency. Muslim women in Sweden are a risk group. *Lakartidningen.* 1996; 93(46): 4153–4155.

43. Schmahl, F.W., Metzler, B. The health risks of occupational stress in Islamic industrial workers during the Ramadan fasting period. *Pol J Occup Med.* 1991; 4(3): 219–228.

44. Stille, A. River of life, river of death. *Science & Spirit.* July–August 2003; 50–55.

45. Pargament, K., Koenig, H., Tarakehswar, N., Hahn, J. Religious struggle as a predictor of mortality among medically ill elderly patients: a two-year longitudinal study. *Archives of Internal Medicine.* 2001; 161(15): 1881–1885.

46. Payne, D. Holy water not always a blessing. *British Medical Journal.* 2001; 322: 190.

47. Hermes Trismegistus. In *Hermetica.* Walter Scott, ed. and trans. (Boulder, Colo.: Hermes House; 1982), 213.

48. Heraclitus. Quoted in Rudolf Steiner, Greek mystery wisdom. In Robert A. McDermott ed. *The Essential Steiner* (San Francisco: Harper & Row, 1984), 189.

49. Thoreau, H.D. Quoted in Auden, W.H., and Kronenberger, L., eds. *The Viking Book of Aphorisms* (New York: Barnes & Noble, 1993), 212.

50. Weil, S. Quoted in Sunbeams. *The Sun.* April 1999, 280: 48.

51. Parton, D. Quoted in Gray, D.R. *Soul Between the Lines* (New York: Avon, 1998), 69.

8. Plants

1. Stillings, D. Human consciousness and vegetable nature. *Healing Island.* Fall 1999; 5: 1–5.

2. Brevoort, P. The booming U.S. botanical market—a new overview. *Herbalgram.* 1998; 44: 33–46. *HerbalGram* is one of the best sources for information about herbs and herbal medicine, published by the American Botanical Council in Austin, TX. For information, contact *HerbalGram*, P. O. 144345,

Austin, TX 78714-4345, tele. 512-926-4900, or visit their Web site at www.herbalgram.org.

3. Oken, B.S., Storzback, D.M., Kaye, J.A. The efficacy of *Ginkgo biloba* on cognitive function in Alzheimer disease. *Archives of Neurology.* 1998: 55: 1409–1415.

4. Watson, L. *Jacobson's Organ* (New York: W.W. Norton, 2000), 193–195.

5. Watson, L., loc. cit., 194.

6. Ausubel, K. ed. *Restoring the Earth: Visionary Solutions from the Bioneers* (Tiburon, Calif.: H.J. Kramer, 2000), 91–102.

7. Ausubel, K., loc. cit., 97.

8. Wu, C. Yin and yang. Western science makes room for Chinese herbal medicine. *Science News.* September 9, 1995; 148: 172–173.

9. Tracy R. Moore, of Monroe, La., is a forest products professional who developed prostate cancer and was treated with conventional chemotherapy at M.D. Anderson Cancer Center in Houston in 1991. During his seven months there, he took advantage of the institution's library and researched his disease. His attention was eventually drawn to China's so-called Tree of Joy, *Camptotheca acuminata.* He and his wife, Ruth Ann, committed their savings to bringing the tree to the United States and growing it in commercial quantities. It has yielded the anticancer drug camptothecin. Moore's inspiring story is described in Petterson, M. The camptothecin tree: harvesting a Chinese anticancer compound in the U.S. *Alternative Therapies in Health and Medicine.* 1996; 1(2): 23–24.

10. Ausubel, K., loc. cit., 112. "Bioneers" stands for biological pioneers. For a decade, Bioneers founder Kenny Ausubel and Nina Simons, his wife and partner, have brought together leading scientists and social visionaries, not to rail at "the establishment," but to exchange intelligent approaches to environmental problems. The annual Bioneers Conference has helped define the modern ecology movement by focusing on pragmatic, original, and scientific solutions. For information about Bioneers, visit www.bioneers.org or call 1-877-BIONEER.

11. Wilson, E.O. *The Diversity of Life* (Cambridge, Mass.: Harvard University Press, 1992), 282–85.

12. Marvel, M.K., Epstein, R.M., Flowers, K., Beckman, H.B. Soliciting the patient's agenda: Have we improved? *Journal of the American Medical Association.* 1999; 281(3): 283–287.

13. Bombeck, E., loc. cit., 40.

14. Grad, B.R. Some biological effects of laying-on of hands: A review of experiments with animals and plants. *Journal of the American Society for Psychical Research.* 1965; 59(vol. A): 95–127.

15. Benor, D.J. *Spiritual Healing* (Southfield, Mich.: Vision, 2002).

16. Dossey, L. The case for nonlocality. *Reinventing Medicine* (San Francisco: HarperSanFrancisco, 1999), 37–84.

17. Hotz, R.L. Seeking the biology of spirituality. *Los Angeles Times.* Sunday, April 26, 1998.

18. Langer, E.J., Rodin, J. The effects of choice and enhanced personality on the aged: A field experience in an institutional setting. *Journal of Personality and Social Psychology.* 1976; 34: 91–98.

19. Take two aspirin and sprout in the morning. *The Sciences.* November/December 1998; 38(6): 7.

20. Chui, G. From chemical weapons to self-preservation methods, plants are apparently savvier than we think. *San Jose Mercury News.* August 10, 1999.

21. *The Oxford Dictionary of Quotations.* Rev. 4th ed., s.v. "Newman, John Henry."

22. Lozoya, X. et al. Survival of cultured plant cells grafted into the subcutaneous tissue of rats (preliminary report). *Archives of Medical Research.* 1995; 26(1): 85–89.

23. Olson, K. O Bioneers! *Utne Reader.* January–February 2001: 28–29.

24. Benyus, J. *Biomimicry: Innovation Inspired by Nature* (New York: William Morrow, 1997).

25. Irwin, A. How man apes animal medicine. www.telegraph.co.uk (accessed December 14, 2000).

26. Ibid.

27. Wu, C. Yin and yang: Western science makes room for Chinese herbal medicine. *Science News.* September 9, 1995; 148: 172–173.

28. Ernst, E. Harmless herbs? a review of the recent literature. *American Journal of Medicine.* 1998; 104: 170–178.

29. Lazarou, J., Pomeranz, B.H., Corey, P.N. Incidence of adverse drug reactions in hospitalized patients. *Journal of the American Medical Association.* 1998; 279(15): 1200–1205.

30. Starfield, B. Is U.S. health really the best in the world? *Journal of the American Medical Association.* 2000; 284(4): 483–485.

31. Mead, N. The endangered herbs. *Utne Reader.* July–August, 1998: 10–11.

32. Ibid.

33. Taxol. *Physician's Desk Reference.* 49th ed. (Montvale, N.J.: Medical Economics Data Production Company, 1995), 682–685.

34. Mead, N., loc. cit., 10–11.

35. Bilger. B. The secret garden. *The Sciences.* January–February 1998, 38–43. Book review of Riddle, J.M. *Eve's Herbs: A History of Contraception and Abortion in the West* (Cambridge, Mass.: Harvard University Press, 1997).

36. Mead, N., loc. cit., 10.

37. Mead, N., loc. cit., 11.

38. Mead, N., loc. cit., 11.

39. Mead, N., loc. cit., 11.

40. Grosso, M. *Soulmaking* (Charlottesville, Va.: Hampton Roads Publishing, Inc., 1997), 108–116.

41. Grosso's experience suggests that New Jersey's moniker, the Garden State, is well deserved.

42. Grosso, M., loc. cit.

9. Bugs

1. Zimmer, C. The healing power of maggots. *Discover.* August 1993; 14(8): 17.

2. Ragavan, C. Back from the brink of hell. *U.S. News & World Report.* July 14, 2003; 135(1): 18–19.

3. McDonald's sued for maggot-infested cheeseburger. Reuters News Service, July 3, 2001. http://dailynews.yahoo.com/h/nm/20010703/od/mcdonalds_dc_2.html (accessed July 3, 2001).

4. Sofer, D. Reach for the leech. *American Journal of Nursing.* 2000; 100(7): 58.

5. Harris, G. Age-old cures, like the maggot, get U.S. hearings. *New York Times.* August 25, 2005: A1.

6. Dunbar, G.K. Notes on the Ngemba tribe of the Central Darling River, Western New South Wales. *Mankind.* 1944; 3: 172–180.

7. Root-Bernstein, R. and M. *Honey, Mud, Maggots, and Other Medical Marvels* (New York: Houghton Mifflin, 1997), 21–30.

8. Root-Bernstein, R. and M., loc. cit., 23.

9. Root-Bernstein, R. and M., loc. cit., 23.

10. Root-Bernstein, R. and M., loc. cit., 25.

11. Sherman, R.A., Hall, M.J.R., Thomas, S. Medicinal maggots: an ancient remedy for some contemporary afflictions. *Annual Review of Entomology.* 2000; 45: 55–81.

12. Root-Bernstein, R. and M., op. cit., 26.

13. Wainwright, M. Maggot therapy—a backwater in the fight against bacterial infection. *Pharmaceutical History* 1988; 30: 19–26.

14. Root-Bernstein, R. and M., op. cit., 28.

15. Blalock, D. Grubby little secret: maggots are neat at fighting infection. *Wall Street Journal.* January 17, 1995: A1, A10.

16. Blalock, D., op. cit., A10.

17. Blalock, D., op. cit., A10.

18. Sherman, R.A., Hall, M.J.R.,Thomas, S., op. cit., 68.

19. Sherman, R.A. Maggot therapy in modern medicine. *Infection and Medicine.* 1998; 15: 651–656.

20. Blalock, D., op. cit., A1.

21. Blalock, D., op. cit., A10.

22. Sherman, R.A., Hall, M.J.R., Thomas, S., op. cit., 72.

23. Sherman, R.A., Hall, M.R.J., Thomas, S., op. cit., 62–70.

24. *World Health Organization Annual Report* (Geneva: WHO, 1998).

25. Sherman, R.A., Hall, M.R.J., Thomas, S., op. cit., 73.

26. Church, J.C.T. The early management of open wounds: shall we use maggots? *East and Central African Journal of Surgery.* 1996; 2: 9–12.

27. Wolff, H., Hansson, C. Larval therapy—an effective method of ulcer debridement. *Clinical and Experimental Dermatology.* 2003; 28(2): 134–137.

28. Adams, S.L. The medicinal leech: a page from the annelids of internal medicine. *Annals of Internal Medicine.* 1988; 1095: 399–405.

29. Adams, S.L., op. cit., 403.

30. Lent, C. New medical and scientific uses of the leech. *Nature.* 1986; 323: 494.

31. Weinstock, M. Gross medicine. Use of leeches and maggots in health care. *Science World.* Oct. 19, 1998. www.findarticles.com (accessed August 13, 2001).

32. Randolph, B.M. The bloodletting controversy in the nineteenth century. *Ann. Med. Hist.* 1935; 7: 177–182.

33. Adams, S.L., op. cit., 400.

34. Ibid.

35. King, J. *Hirudo medicinalis.* In *The American Dispensatory.* 8th ed. (Cincinnati: Wilstach, Baldwin & Co., 1870), 424–426.

36. Adams, S.L., op. cit., 403.

37. Ibid.

38. Adams, S.L., op. cit., 402.

39. Harder, B. Creepy-crawly care: Maggots move into mainstream medicine. *Science News.* October 23, 2004; 166: 266–268.

40. Hartig, G.K., Connor, N.P., et al. Comparing a mechanical device with medicinal leeches for treating venous congestion. *Otolaryngology-Head and Neck Surgery.* 2003; 129: 556–564. dx.doi.org/10.1016/S0194-5998(03)01587-0 (accessed November 1, 2004).

41. Michalsen, A. Effectiveness of leech therapy in osteoarthritis of the knee: A randomized, controlled trial. *Annals of Internal Medicine.* 2003; 139: 724–730. www.annals.org/cgi/content/abstract/139/9/724 (accessed November 1, 2004).

42. Lauck, J.E. *The Voice of the Infinite in the Small: Revisioning the Insect-Human Connection* (Mill Spring, N.C.: Swan Raven & Co., 1998), 50.

43. Taylor, R. *Butterflies in My Stomach or: Insects in Human Nutrition* (Santa Barbara: Woodbridge Press, 1975).

44. Lauck, J.E., op. cit., 49.

45. Elmer, G.W. Probiotics: "living drugs." *American Journal of Health Systems Pharmacy.* 2001; 58(12): 1101–1109.

46. Ready, T. Good germs, bad germs. *Utne Reader.* November–December, 2001; 108: 26–28.

47. Bugs fight terrorism. *New York Times Magazine.* October 24, 2004: 49.

48. Dickerson, J. Tarantula venom could be a new source for healing. *USA Today.* December 15, 2004: 7D.

49. Van Kolfschooten, F. Diet of worms can cure bowel disease. *New Scientist.* April 6, 2004. www.newscientist.com/news/print.jsp?id=ns99994852 (accessed November 1, 2004).

50. Diet of worms solves gut problems. BBC News Online. news.bbc.co.uk/1 /hi/health/412142.stm (accessed November 1, 2004).

51. *Bartlett's Familiar Quotations.* 16th ed., s.v. "Bierce."

10. Unhappiness

1. Engel, G.L. Sudden and rapid death during psychological stress: folk lore or folk wisdom? *Annals of Internal Medicine.* 1971; 74: 771–782.

2. Denker, D. *Sisters on the Bridge of Fire* (Los Angeles: Burning Gate Press; 1993), 58.

3. Csikszentmihalyi, M. *The Evolving Self* (New York: HarperCollins, 1993).

4. Ibid., 35–37.

5. Watts, A. *Odyssey of Aldous Huxley.* Original Live Recordings on Comparative Philosophy (San Anselmo, Calif.: The Electronic University, 1995).

6. Russell, B. Quoted in Sunbeams. *The Sun.* 1994; 217: 40.

7. Csikszentmihalyi, M., op. cit., 35–37.

8. Csikszentmihalyi, M., op. cit., 36.

9. Csikszentmihalyi, M., op. cit., 36. *The World Times,* a nationally distributed newspaper published in Santa Fe, N.M., is a refreshing contrast. It publishes only good news.

10. Csikszentmihalyi, M., op. cit., 7.

11. Bulger, R.J. Narcissus, Pogo, and Lew Thomas' wager. *Journal of the American Medical Association.* 1981; 245: 1450–1454.

12. Lanier, J. From having a mystical experience to becoming a mystic. *ReVision.* 1989; 12 (1): 41–44. Reprint and epilogue.

13. Ibid.

14. Source unknown. Quoted in Syfransky, S., ed. *Sunbeams: A Book of Quotations* (Berkeley: North Atlantic, 1990), 45.

15. Goldberg, N. *Wild Mind: Living the Writer's Life* (New York: Bantam, 1990).

16. Douglass, F. In Sunbeams. *The Sun.* 1995; 231: 40.

11. Nothing

1. Dossey, L. The great wait: in praise of doing nothing. *Alternative Therapies in Health and Medicine.* 1996; 2(6): 8–14.

2. Weil, A. *Spontaneous Healing* (New York: Alfred A. Knopf, 1995), 4–5.

3. O'Regan, B., Hirshberg, C. *Spontaneous Remission: An Annotated Bibliography* (Sausalito, Calif.: Institute of Noetic Sciences, 1993), 3.

4. Ayres, R.C.S., Robertson, D.A.F., Dewbury, K.C., Millward-Sadler, G.H., Smith, C.L. Spontaneous regression of hepatocellular carcinoma. *Gut.* 1990; 31(6): 722–724.

5. O'Regan, B., Hirshberg, C., op. cit., 7.

6. Thomas, L. *The Youngest Science: Notes of a Medicine Watcher* (New York: Viking Press, 1983), 205.

7. Hirshberg, C., Barasch, M.I. *Remarkable Recovery* (New York: Riverhead, 1995), 332–333.

8. McLaughlin, L. Obese kids. *Time.* March 11, 2002: 86.

9. Weinberger, M., Oddone, E.Z., Henderson, W.G. Does increased access to primary care reduce hospital admissions? Veterans Affairs Cooperative Study Group on Primary Care and Hospital Readmission. *N. Eng. J. Med.* 1996; 334(22): 1441–1447.

10. Welch, H.G. Quoted in Medical study blasts a theory. Associated Press release. May 29, 1996.

11. CNN Headline News. April 15, 1996.

12. Lao Tsu. *Tao Te Ching.* Feng, G.F., and English, J., trans. (New York: Alfred A. Knopf, 1972), 22.

13. Lao Tsu, ibid., 96.

14. Jung, C.G. Commentary. In Wilhelm, R. *The Secret of the Golden Flower* (New York: Harcourt Brace Jovanovich, 1962), 91.

15. Huron, A. Coffee, tool of the man. *Utne Reader.* May–June 2002; No. 111: 39.

16. Nedzel, R. A truly outstanding article. *Utne Reader.* May–June 2002; No. 111: 33–34.

17. Garfield, S. *Mauve: How One Man Invented a Color that Changed the World* (New York: W. W. Norton, 2000), 88.

18. *Webster's New World Dictionary,* 2nd College ed.

19. Quindlen, A. Doing nothing is something. *Newsweek.* May 13, 2002; 139(19): 76.

20. Dossey, B.M. *Florence Nightingale: Mystic, Visionary, Healer* (Springhouse, Pa.: Springhouse, 2000).

21. Nightingale, F. *Notes From Devotional Authors of the Middle Ages: Collected, Chosen, and Freely Translated by Florence Nightingale.* London: BL Add. Mss. 45841: ff 1–87. Unpublished manuscript.

22. Huxley, A. *The Perennial Philosophy* (New York: Harper & Row, 1945), 21.

23. *Bartlett's Familiar Quotations,* 16th ed., s.v. "Twain, Mark."

24. Huxley, A., op. cit., 218–219.

25. See note 23.

26. Castaneda, C. *Tales of Power* (New York: Simon & Schuster, 1974), 33.

27. Satprem. Quoted in Walsh, R., Vaughan, F. Towards an integrative psychology of well-being. *Beyond Health and Normality: Explorations of Exceptional Psychological Well-being.* Walsh, R., Shapiro, D.H., eds. (New York: Van Nostrand Reinhold Company, 1983), 403.

28. *Bartlett's Familiar Quotations,* 16th ed., s.v. "Lao Tze."

29. St. John of the Cross. Quoted in Huxley, A., *The Perennial Philosophy* (New York: Harper & Row, 1945), 218.

30. Carpenter, E. Quoted in Walsh, R., and Vaughan, F., Towards an integrative psychology of well-being. In *Beyond Health and Normality: Explorations of Exceptional Psychological Well-being.* Walsh, R., and Shapiro, D.H., eds. (New York: Van Nostrand Reinhold Company, 1983), 399–400.

31. Huxley, A., op. cit., 223–224.

32. *The Oxford Dictionary of Quotations.* Revised ed., s.v. "Blake, William."

33. Coomaraswamy, A.K. *Hinduism and Buddhism* (New York: Philosophical Library, 1996), 28.

34. Maharshi, R. Quoted in Wilber, K., *The Spectrum of Consciousness* (Wheaton, Ill.: Theosophical Publishing House, 1977), 76.

35. Stace, W.T. *Mysticism and Philosophy* (London: Macmillan, 1960), 85–86.

36. Russell, P. *From Science to God: The Mystery of Consciousness and the Meaning of Light* (Pre-publication edition; 2000), 77.

37. Russell, P., op. cit., 78.

38. Underhill, E. *Mysticism* (New York: E.P. Dutton, 1961).

39. Smith, H. *The Religions of Man* (New York: Harper & Row, 1986), 132.

40. Ibid.

41. Dossey, B.M., op. cit.

42. Wallace, A. The Potential of emptiness: Vacuum states in physics and consciousness. *Network.* 2001; 77: 21–25.

43. Dainton, B. The gaze of consciousness. *Journal of Consciousness Studies.* 2002; 9(2): 31–48.

44. Allen, J.R., Pfefferbaum, B., Hammond, D., Speed, L. A disturbed child's use of a public event. *Psychiatry.* 2000 Summer; 63(2): 208–213.

45. Forstl, H., Beats, B. Charles Bonnet's description of Cotard's delusion and reduplicative paramnesia in an elderly patient (1788). *Br. J. Psychiatry.* 1992; 161: 133–134.

46. Pearn, J., Gardner-Thorpe, C. Jules Cotard (1840–1889): his life and the unique syndrome which bears his name. *Neurology.* 2002; 14(58): 1400–1403.

47. Warren, N. The quick and the undead. *Fortean Times.* 2002; 159: 25.

48. Puthoff, H.E. Searching for the universal matrix in metaphysics. *Research News and Opportunities in Science and Theology.* April 2002; 2(8): 22, 32.

49. Targ, R., Puthoff, H. *Mind-Reach. Scientists Look at Psychic Ability* (New York: Delta, 1977).

50. Puthoff, H., op. cit., 32.

51. Rauscher, E.A., Targ, R. The speed of thought: Investigation of a complex space-time metric to describe psychic phenomena. *Journal of Scientific Exploration.* 2001; 15(3): 331–354.

52. Jahn, R.G., Dunne, B.J. A modular model of mind/matter manifestations (M^5). *Journal of Scientific Exploration.* 2001; 15(3): 299–329.

53. Josephson, B., Pallikara-Villas, F. 1991. Biological untilization of quantum nonlocality. *Foundations of Physics.* 21: 197–207.

54. Clarke, C.J.S. The nonlocality of mind. *Journal of Consciousness Studies.* 1995; 2(3): 231–40.

55. Sheldrake, R. *A New Science of Life: The Hypothesis of Formative Causation* (Blond and Briggs; London: 1981).

56. Puthoff, H., op. cit., 32.

57. Starfield, B. Is U.S. health really the best in the world? *Journal of the American Medical Association.* 2000; 284(4): 483–485.

58. Hrobjartsson, A., Gotzsche, P.C. Is the placebo powerless? An analysis of clinical trials comparing placebo with no treatment. *New England Journal of Medicine.* 2001; 344(21): 1594–1602.

59. Kolata, G. Researchers debunk placebo effect, saying it's only a myth. *The New York Times* on the Web. www.nytimes.com/2001/05/23/health/23CND-PLAC.html?pagewanted=print (accessed May 23, 2001).

60. Hotz, R.L. Healing body by fakery. www.latimes.com/news/science/la000012483feb18.story?coll=la%2Dnews%2Dscience (accessed February 19, 2002).

61. Haseltine, E. The greatest unanswered questions of physics. *Discover.* 2002; 23(2): 37–42.

62. Barrow, J.D. *The Book of Nothing: Vacuums, Voids, and the Latest ideas about the Origins of the Universe* (New York: Pantheon, 2000), 265.

63. Ibid.

64. Greene, B. *The Elegant Universe* (New York: Vintage, 2000).

65. Turner, M.S. More than meets the eye. *The Sciences.* 2000; 40(6): 32–37.

66. Turner, M.S., op. cit., 37.

67. Barrow, J., op. cit., 244.

68. Barrow, J., op. cit., 300.

69. Barrow, J., op. cit., 301.

70. *Bartlett's Familiar Quotations,* 16th ed., s.v. "Allen, Woody."

71. Folger, T. Does the universe exist if we're not looking? *Discover.* June 2002; 23(6): 44–48.

72. Folger, T., op. cit., 48.

73. Dossey, L. The case for nonlocality. *Reinventing Medicine* (San Francisco: HarperSanFrancisco, 1999), 37–84.

12. Voices

1. Inglis, B. *Natural and Supernatural: A History of the Paranormal* (Bridport, Dorset, U.K.: Prism Press, 1992), 56.

2. Schneider, W. Bush's father figure. American Enterprise Institute for Public Policy Research. www.aei.org/news/filter.,newsID.20397/news_detail.asp April 30, 2004 (accessed December 8, 2004).

3. Socrates. Quoted in Inglis, B. *Natural and Supernatural: A History of the Paranormal* (Bridport, Dorset, U.K.: Prism Press, 1992), 57.

4. Homer. *The Iliad.* Quoted in Fox, R.L. *Pagans and Christians* (San Francisco: Harper & Row/Perennial Library, 1986), 418.

5. Inglis, B., op. cit., 55.

6. Le Goff, J. *The Birth of Purgatory.* Arthur Goldhammer, trans. (Chicago: University of Chicago Press, 1984), 82.

7. Plutarch. Quoted in Inglis, B. *Natural and Supernatural: A History of the Paranormal* (Bridport, Dorset, U.K.: Prism Press, 1992), 56.

8. Barnum, B.S. *Mystic Encounters: The Door Ajar.* Forthcoming.

9. Barnum, B. Expanded consciousness: nurses' experiences. *Nursing Outlook.* 1989; 37(6): 260–266.

10. Barnum, B. op. cit., 264.

11. Rees, W.D. The bereaved and their hallucinations. In *Bereavement: Its Psychosocial Aspects.* Schoenberg, B., Kutscher, A.H., Carr, A.C., eds. (New York: Columbia University Press, 1975).

12. Romme, M., Escher, S. *Making Sense of Voices* (London: Mind Publications, 2000).

13. Garety, P. Book review of *Making Sense of Voices. Psychiatric Bulletin.* 2001; 25: 406–407.

14. Hearing voices "can be health." news.bbc.co.uk/1/hi/health/963545.stm. October 10, 2000 (accessed December 8, 2004).

15. Jaynes, J. *The Origin of Consciousness in the Breakdown of the Bicameral Mind* (New York: Houghton Mifflin, 1976).

16. Hastings, A. *With the Tongues of Men and Angels: A Study of Channeling* (Orlando, Fl.: Holt, Rinehart and Winston, 1991), 122.

17. Woodward shares war secrets. Interview on *60 Minutes.* www.cbsnews.com/ stories/2004/04/15/60minutes/main612067.shtml (accessed July 19, 2004).

18. Bloom, L. Religious leaders criticize Bush administration over Iraq. United Methodist Church Web site. May 4, 2004. www.umc.org/interior.asp?ptid= 17&mid=4544 (accessed July 20, 2004).

19. Saba, P.R., Keshavan, M.S. Musical hallucinations and musical imagery: prevalence and phenomenology in schizophrenic patients. *Psychopathology.* 1997; 30(4): 185–190.

20. Rivenburg, R. Catchy tunes that get lodged in brain create cognitive itch. *The Honolulu Advertiser.* October 15, 2001. www.honoluluadvertiser.com (accessed October 15, 2001). This article is based on: Kellaris, J.J. Identifying properties of tunes that get "stuck in your head": toward a theory of cognitive itch. In Heckler, S.E. and Shapiro, S. eds. Proceedings of the Society for Consumer Psychology Winter 2001 Conference, Scottsdale, Ariz.

21. Ibid.

22. Azuonye, I.O. A difficult case: diagnosis made by hallucinatory voices. *British Medical Journal.* 1997; 315: 1685–1686.

23. Tomlin, L. Quoted in www.brainyquote.com/quotes/quotes/l/lilytomlin 141908.html (accessed July 17, 2004).

24. Barrett, T.R., Etheridge, J.B. Verbal hallucinations in normals, I: People who hear "voices." *Applied Cognitive Psychology.* 1992; 6: 379–387.

25. Barrett, T.R. Verbal hallucinations in normals, II: Self-reported imagery vividness. *Personality and Individual Differences.* 1993; 15: 61–67.

26. Barrett, T.R., Etheridge, J.B. Verbal hallucinations in normals, III: Dysfunctional personality correlates. *Personality and Individual Differences.* 1994; 16: 57–62.

27. Schrödinger, F. In Dossey, L. *Recovering the Soul: A Scientific and Spiritual Search* (New York: Bantam, 1989), 125–137.

28. Hastings, A., op. cit., 121, 185–194.

29. Dossey, B.M. *Florence Nightingale: Mystic, Visionary, Healer* (Springhouse, Pa.: Springhouse, 2000).

30. Alschuler, A.S. Recognizing inner teachers—inner voices throughout history. *Gnosis Magazine.* Fall 1987; 5: 8–12.

31. Alschuler, A.S. Inner teachers and transcendent education. In Rao, K.R. ed., *Cultivating Consciousness: Enhancing Human Potential, Wellness, and Healing* (Westport, CT: Praeger, 1993), 181–193.

32. Alschuler, A.S. Inner voices and inspired lives through the ages. In Thayer, S.J. and Nathanson, L.S., eds., *Interview with an Angel: Our World, Our Selves, Our Destiny* (Gillette, NJ: Edin Books, 1996), 1–62.

33. Sylvia, C. *A Change of Heart: A Memoir.* With William Novak (Boston: Little Brown, 1997).

34. Dossey, L. *Recovering the Soul* (New York: Bantam, 1989): 1–11.

35. Von Franz, M.L. *On Divination and Synchronicity: The Psychology of Meaningful Chance* (Toronto: Inner City Books, 1980), 39.

36. Ibid.

13. Mystery

1. These are generalizations, of course. All good surgeons are also interested in knowing, and all gifted internists are also devoted to doing.

2. James, W. *The Will to Believe* (New York: Dover, 1956).

3. Dossey, L. What's in a name? *Alternative Therapies in Health and Medicine.* 1999; 5(5): 12–17, 100–102.

4. Hurdle, J. Lose weight, stay active, prevent Alzheimer's—Studies. Reuter's Online. www.reuters.com. July 19, 2004 (accessed July 20, 2004).

5. Hague, R. The pull of mystery. www.writersdigest.com/articles/hague_mystery.asp (accessed December 30, 2004).

6. Thomas, L. Quoted in Albert J. Wallace Stegner (1909–1993). www.cateweb.org/CA_Authors/Stegner.html (accessed January 1, 2005).

7. Hazleton, L. *Mary: A Flesh-and-Blood Biography of the Virgin Mother* (New York: Bloomsbury, 2004), 123.

8. Hall, R. Quoted in Mystery.en.thinkexist.com/quotes/ (accessed December 10, 2004).

9. Asimov, I. Quoted in *Journal of the American Medical Association.* 2004; 291(1): 2350.

10. Bacon, F. Quoted in Eiseley, L., *The Man Who Saw Through Time* (New York: Scribner's, 1961), 115.

11. Huxley, A. Quoted in Murray, N., *Aldous Huxley: A Biography* (New York: Thomas Dunne/St. Martin's Press, 2002), 174.

12. Unsoeld, W. Wilderness and the sacred. *Green Screens.* June 1999. www.olywa.net/speech/june99/willi.html (accessed December 14, 2004).

13. Otto, R. *The Idea of the Holy.* Harvey, J.W., trans. (New York: Oxford University Press, 1958).

14. Unsoeld, W. Quoted in Willie Unsoeld: brief biography and quotes. www.wilderdom.com/Unsoeld.htm (accessed December 29, 2004).

15. Stegner, W. *The Wilderness Letter,* written to the Outdoor Recreation Resources Review Commission, 1962, and subsequently in *The Sound of Mountain Water* (New York: Doubleday, 1969). Also www.wilderness.org/Library/Documents/Wilderness_Quotes.cfm (accessed December 29, 2004).

16. Shepard, Jr., T. *John F. Kennedy, Man of the Sea* (New York: Morrow, 1965), 23.

17. Zappa, F. Quoted in the big list o' Frank. sam.hochberg.com/zappa.html (accessed January 3, 2004).

18. Van Wagenen, R. Wilderness as metaphor for mystery. www.hupc.org/Archive/newsletters/Dec.%201999/metaphor.htm (accessed December 10, 2004.

19. May, R. Wonder and ethics in therapy. www.nfgcc.org/47.htm (accessed December 11, 2004).

14. Miracles

1. Hirshberg, C., Barasch, M.I. *Remarkable Recovery* (New York: Riverhead; 1995: 117–24.

2. Klaus, R. *Rita's Story* (Cape Cod: Paraclete Press, 1993). Klaus's story is available on video and audio cassettes, "Healed from Multiple Sclerosis," at www.catholicfocus.com.

3. Hirshberg, C., Barasch, M.I., op. cit., 122.

4. Ibid.

5. Ibid.

6. Ibid., 37–38.

7. Ibid.

8. Jones, T. The saint and Ann O'Neill. *The Washington Post,* Sunday, April 3, 1994, Style section, F1–F5. Cited in Hirshberg, C., Barasch, M.I., op. cit., 137.

9. Bloom, H.D.G., Richardson, W.W., Harries, E.J. Natural history of untreated breast cancer. 1805–1933. *British Medical Journal.* 1962; 2: 213–221.

10. Challis, G.B., Stam, H.J. The spontaneous regression of cancer: a review of cases from 1900 to 1987. *Acta Oncologica.* 1990; 29 (5): 545–550.

11. Ayres, R.C.S. Spontaneous regression of hepatocellular carcinoma. *Gut.* 1990; 31 (6): 722–724.

12. Hirshberg, C., Barasch, M.I., op. cit., 137.

13. Osler, Sir W. The faith that heals. *British Medical Journal.* June 18, 1910: 1471.

14. Dowling, S.J. Lourdes cures and their medical assessment. *Journal of the Royal Society of Medicine.* 1984; 77: 634–8.

15. Dowling, S.J., op. cit., 634.

16. Dowling, S.J., op. cit., 636.

17. Dowling, S.J., op. cit., 637.

18. Dowling, S.J., op. cit., 638.

19. Most Americans believe in miracles. *Newsweek* poll. May 1, 2000. www.newsweek.com. See also Woodward, K. *The Book of Miracles* (New York: Touchstone, 2001).

20. Yankelovich Partners. Survey of family physicians presented at the American Academy of Family Physicians Annual meeting, October 1996, as reported in *Parade Magazine,* Dec. 1, 1996.

21. Pfenninger. J.L., Fowler, G.C. *Procedures for Primary Care Physicians* (St. Louis: Mosby, 1994).

22. Guernsey, D. My prayer. *Town & Country.* September 2002: 164.

23. Shapiro, S.L. Spontaneous regression of cancer. *Eye, Ear, Nose, Throat Monthly.* 1967; 46(10): 1306–1310.

24. Ibid.

25. O'Regan, B. Healing, remission and miracle cures. *Institute of Noetic Sciences Special Report.* May 1987: 1–14.

26. O'Regan, B. op. cit., 11.

27. Dossey, L. Saints and sinners, health and illness. *Healing Words* (San Francisco: HarperSanFrancisco; 1993), 13–36.

28. *Webster's New World Dictionary,* 2nd College ed.

29. Voltaire. Quoted in Michael Grosso, Miracles: illusions, natural events, or divine interventions. *Journal of Religion and Psychical Research.* 1997; 20(4): 187.

30. Grosso, M. Miracles: illusions, natural events, or divine interventions. *Journal of Religion and Psychical Research.* 1997; 20(4): 187.

31. Freud, S. *Complete Psychological Works,* Standard Edition (London: Hogarth Press, 1955).

32. Grosso, M., op. cit., 187.

33. Cary, J. Believing. *Parabola.* 1997; XXII(4): 34–36.

34. Wertenbaker, C. Laws, miracles, and science. *Parabola.* 1997; XXII(4): 51–55.

35. *The Persian Mystics: The Invocations of Sheikh 'Abdullâh Ansâri of Herat.* Sardar Sri Jogendra Singh, trans. (London: John Murray, 1939).

36. Cornwell, B. *Sharpe's Company* (New York: Penguin, 1982), 151.

37. Grosso, M. *Soulmaking* (Charlottesville, VA: Hampton Roads, 1997), 53, 200–201.

38. Grosso, M. Miracles: Illusions, natural events, or divine intervention? *The Journal of Religion and Psychical Research.* 1997; 20(1): 2–18.

39. Grosso, M., op. cit., 9.

40. Einstein, A. Quotes of Albert Einstein. physics.augustana.edu/einstein. html (accessed April 20, 2005).

41. Bockris, J. O'M. Book review of Sagan, C., *The Demon-Haunted World* (New York: Random House, 1995). *Journal of Scientific Exploration.* 1997; 11 (4): 559–563.

42. King, M.B. Consciousness at the zero point. *Light of Consciousness.* 1998; 10 (1): 28.

Index

ABOUT THE AUTHOR

LARRY DOSSEY, MD, is a former internist and chief of staff of Medical City Dallas Hospital and former co-chair of the Panel on Mind/Body Interventions, National Center for Complementary and Alternative Medicine, National Institutes of Health. He is the executive editor of *Explore: The Journal of Science and Healing* and the author of ten books on the role of consciousness and spirituality in healing, including the *New York Times* bestseller *Healing Words: The Power of Prayer and the Practice of Medicine*. Dr. Dossey lives in Santa Fe with his wife, award-winning author Barbara Montgomery Dossey, PhD, RN. His Web site is www.dosseydossey.com.